100 MENTAL HEALTH JOURNALING PROMPTS

JOURNALING PROMPTS SERIES

RICHARD FRENCH

ALSO BY RICHARD FRENCH

NON FICTION

The Art of Journaling

Write Your Way

Advanced Pattern Recognition

The Year End Reflection Guide

100 Self-Discovery Journaling Prompts

100 Mental Health Journaling Prompts

Revelation Explained: Verse by Verse

Proverbs for Profit

Daniel as a Blueprint for Navigating Ethical Dilemmas (2nd Edition)

FICTION

The Convergence: Broken Magic

The Convergence: Restoration

Indie Pen Press

Turning Dreams into Best Sellers

Indie Pen Press
Seattle, Washington USA
IndiePenPress.com

First Edition: July 2025

Paperback ISBN: 979-8-9991846-4-1

Library of Congress Control Number: 2025941651

CONTENTS

PREFACE: THE SCIENCE BEHIND MENTAL HEALTH AND WRITING

You know that feeling when you discover something simple that changes everything? That's exactly what happened when scientists started paying serious attention to therapeutic writing. People have been pouring their hearts onto paper for centuries, but we finally understand why this practice can be such a game-changer for anxiety, depression, stress, and just about every emotional challenge life throws our way.

WHEN WORDS BECOME MEDICINE

Here's a story that might surprise you. Back in 1986, psychology professor James Pennebaker had a simple idea. He asked college students to write about their deepest thoughts and feelings for just fifteen minutes a day, four days in a row. The results? These students visited the health center half as often over the next six months compared to students who wrote about everyday topics like their shoes. Their immune systems got stronger, stress levels dropped, and they gained clearer insight into their lives.

You might think this was just a lucky coincidence, but here's the thing: over the past forty years, scientists have tested this with thousands of people across 146 different studies. The pattern holds. When Dr. Joshua Smyth crunched the numbers from thirteen major studies, he found that people who did therapeutic writing were doing better than about 70% of people who didn't write at all. That's not a small difference.

When you write about something that's bothering you, something fascinating happens in your brain. Your scattered thoughts and overwhelming feelings start organizing themselves into something that makes sense. Brain scans show us that handwriting lights up more areas of your brain than typing does, connecting the parts that handle emotions with the parts that solve problems. Your brain literally learns to handle difficult feelings more skillfully.

WHAT THE NUMBERS REALLY TELL US

The science reveals some clear patterns about when therapeutic writing helps most. People working through trauma see the biggest changes. When proper safety measures are in place, about 8 out of 10 people show meaningful improvement. If you're dealing with anxiety, you might see roughly 1 in 10 of your symptoms ease up. That might sound small, but imagine feeling 10% less anxious every day. It adds up to real relief.

Depression is trickier. Writing alone doesn't cure depression, but when you combine it with therapy or other treatment, it can make everything work better. Gratitude writing, for example, helps about 1 in 5 people feel noticeably better about their lives.

Dr. Pennebaker's team figured out the sweet spot: 15 to 20 minutes of writing, three or four times over a few days or weeks. Write for less time and your emotions don't have space to process. Write for too long and you can get overwhelmed. The magic happens when you're alone in a place where you feel safe to be completely honest.

HOW YOUR BODY JOINS THE HEALING

Here's what really amazed researchers: therapeutic writing doesn't just help your mind, it helps your whole body. People who write regularly handle stress better. Their heart rate stays steadier during tough times. They get sick less often and even respond better to vaccines.

Brain scans show that people who write therapeutically develop stronger connections between the emotional and logical parts of their brains. This is why writing can turn overwhelming feelings into thoughts you can actually work with. Your brain rewires itself to be better at handling whatever life brings.

THE DIGITAL AGE OF HEALING

Technology is opening exciting new doors for therapeutic writing. In 2024, researchers tested AI-powered journaling apps and got results that blew everyone away. People using smart writing prompts improved at rates that matched traditional therapy. About 8 out of 10 people saw their depression symptoms improve, and similar numbers found relief from anxiety.

But here's what matters: technology works best when it includes real human support for crisis situations and clear limits about what apps can and can't do. No app can replace the wisdom of a skilled therapist when you're dealing with serious mental health challenges.

WHO BENEFITS AND WHEN

Therapeutic writing isn't a magic bullet for everyone. Some people have trouble identifying their emotions, which makes expressive writing feel frustrating rather than helpful. If you're experiencing hallucinations or delusions, you need professional support, not self-guided writing. And if you've been through trauma in the past six months, work with a trained therapist rather than trying to process it alone through writing.

Culture matters too. Most of these studies focused on people from Western backgrounds where sharing personal feelings is encouraged. If you come from a culture that values community over individual expression, you might need to adapt these approaches to feel right for you.

The clearest finding from all this research? Therapeutic writing works best alongside professional treatment, not instead of it. When you combine writing with therapy or medication, both work better. Writing becomes a bridge between your therapy sessions and real life, giving you a tool that's always available when you need support.

YOUR SAFE PATH FORWARD

This book turns all these scientific discoveries into practical tools you can use safely. Every suggestion is grounded in evidence from cognitive behavioral therapy, mindfulness practices, and trauma-informed care. The writing prompts are designed to give you maximum benefit while keeping you emotionally safe.

The pages ahead offer you a path toward better mental health that's backed by solid science. The research helps us understand why these practices work, but your personal experience will be entirely your own. Trust both the evidence and your own wisdom as you explore these tools.

Your journey starts with the simple courage to meet yourself honestly on the page, supported by decades of research showing how words really can heal the mind.

INTRODUCTION: THE HEALING JOURNEY OF MENTAL WELLNESS

You know that moment when you're carrying so much inside and you just need somewhere safe to put it all? That's exactly what therapeutic writing offers you. People have been finding healing through putting pen to paper for centuries, working through trauma, calming anxiety, lifting depression, and discovering strength they didn't know they had.

Let me tell you about some remarkable people who found their way through writing. Anne Frank, hiding in an attic during the Holocaust, poured her heart into her diary. Those pages weren't just keeping track of what happened each day. They became her lifeline to hope when everything felt hopeless. Maya Angelou wrote her way back to speaking after trauma stole her voice as a child. Virginia Woolf captured the ups and downs of what we now understand as bipolar disorder, leaving us a map of how the mind works when it's struggling.

Here's what I find so beautiful about their stories: none of them were therapists or mental health professionals. They were just people, like you and me, who discovered that something magical happens when you meet yourself honestly on the page. Their journals became the friend who never judged, the safe space that was always available, the place where they could work through everything from everyday worries to life-changing losses.

WHAT WE NOW KNOW ABOUT WHY WRITING HEALS

Here's something that might surprise you: scientists have now proven what Anne Frank and Maya Angelou knew in their hearts. When thousands of people have tried therapeutic writing in carefully designed studies, about 7 out of 10 feel better than people who don't write at all. That might not sound huge, but imagine if 7 out of 10 times you felt anxious, you had a tool that genuinely helped. That's life-changing.

And here's the best part: you don't need perfect grammar or beautiful handwriting or profound insights. You just need to show up with honesty. Free-form journaling can definitely help, but when you have gentle prompts guiding you, the healing happens faster and goes deeper. That's exactly what this book offers you. Every suggestion here comes from decades of work with people who've walked through anxiety, depression, trauma, and all kinds of emotional challenges.

Dr. Pennebaker figured out the sweet spot years ago: just 15 to 20 minutes of writing, three or four times over a few days or weeks. The people in his studies visited the doctor half as often over the next six months. Brain scans now show us why this works so beautifully. When you write about what's troubling you, your brain literally builds stronger bridges between the part that feels and the part that thinks. You get better at handling whatever life throws your way.

WHAT YOU CAN REALISTICALLY EXPECT

Let me be completely honest with you: therapeutic writing isn't going to fix everything overnight. What it will do is give you a reliable, gentle tool that you can use anytime, anywhere, for absolutely free. Think of it as one really good friend in your support network. For some challenges like trauma and anxiety, about 8 out of 10 people find meaningful relief when they follow safe writing practices. Depression can be trickier, but writing becomes much more powerful when you combine it with other support like therapy or medication.

Your background matters too. Most studies have included people from Western cultures where talking about feelings is pretty normal. If you come from a family or culture where sharing emotions feels uncomfortable, you might need to adapt these approaches to feel right for you. And different techniques work better at different life stages. The beautiful thing is how accessible this practice is. You can do it in your pajamas at 2 AM if that's when you need it most.

HOW THIS BOOK BECOMES YOUR GUIDE

I've organized these prompts to meet you exactly where you are right now in your mental health journey. Imagine them as different trails through a peaceful garden, each one designed for what you need most.

Daily Foundation Prompts are like gentle morning check-ins with yourself. These seven rotating prompts help you notice the emotional weather of your day, spot stress patterns before they build up, and reconnect with your own strength. They take just 10 to 15 minutes, perfect for those quiet moments when you want to touch base with how you're really doing.

Weekly Reflection Prompts help you zoom out and see the bigger picture. These thirteen prompts reveal patterns you might miss day by day. Maybe you'll discover that Sunday evenings always make you anxious, or that certain friends consistently lift your mood. These insights become gold for managing your mental health.

Monthly Deep Dives are for when you're ready to explore the deeper currents of your emotional life. These fifteen prompts invite you to look at core beliefs, long-term patterns, and the bigger story of your healing journey. Perfect for those times when you want to make thoughtful changes that really support your well-being.

Situational Prompts are like having a wise friend available exactly when life gets tough. Sixty-five prompts designed for specific challenges: when anxiety strikes, when depression settles in, when stress feels overwhelming, or when you're rebuilding after something difficult. Each set includes safety guidelines to keep you emotionally secure.

MEET YOUR COMPANIONS ON THIS JOURNEY

I want you to meet two people who've walked this path before you. Sarah is a 34-year-old graphic designer who felt like her perfectionism and anxiety were taking over her life. Work deadlines sent her into spirals, and she was exhausting herself trying to make everything perfect. James, a 42-year-old teacher, found himself in the fog of depression after his divorce. He felt disconnected from everyone, convinced he was just bringing people down.

Here's what I love about their stories: they're real. These are composites of actual people who've used therapeutic writing to transform their lives. Neither Sarah nor James woke up one morning completely healed. Instead, they discovered something gentler and more sustainable. By consistently meeting themselves with kindness on the page, they developed deeper self-understanding, better ways of coping, and most importantly, a friendlier relationship with their own minds.

Sarah learned that her perfectionism was actually her anxiety wearing a disguise. Through gentle writing prompts, she began to see the difference between caring about quality and wearing herself out with impossible standards. James discovered that his journal became the safe friend he could always turn to. Writing helped him see his own resilience and develop practical ways to manage the tough days.

KEEPING YOU SAFE EVERY STEP OF THE WAY

Before we dive in, I need to share something important about safety. Therapeutic writing is incredibly powerful, which means we need to be thoughtful about when it's the right fit and when you might need additional support.

Some people find it really hard to identify emotions, which can make expressive writing feel frustrating rather than helpful. If you're experiencing hallucinations or having trouble telling what's real, you need professional support right alongside any writing practice. And if you've been through trauma in the past six months, please work with a trained therapist rather than trying to process those big experiences alone through writing.

Every chapter includes clear guidance about when to reach out for extra help and how writing can work beautifully alongside therapy or medication. I've marked all the warning signs that mean it's time to call for professional support, plus I'll give you crisis resources and backup plans.

Think of these safety guidelines as guardrails that keep you secure while you explore and heal.

YOUR PATH FORWARD STARTS HERE

Your mental health journey belongs entirely to you. Some days you might have profound insights that shift everything. Other days might bring quiet observations or feelings that seem unclear. All of these experiences matter and serve your healing.

You're not trying to reach some perfect destination or find all the answers. You're building a kinder, more understanding relationship with your own mental health through honest reflection.

Thousands of people have used these prompts to better understand their anxiety, depression, stress, and other challenges. They've found bridges through difficult times and tools for staying well during peaceful periods. Most importantly, they've realized they're not alone in their struggles and that healing really is possible, one gentle reflection at a time.

As you turn to the next page, remember something beautiful: every single person who has found healing through writing started exactly where you are right now. They had curiosity, courage, and willingness to meet themselves honestly on the page. Your journey toward mental wellness through therapeutic writing begins whenever you feel ready to begin.

ONE
BEGINNING YOUR JOURNEY: A GUIDE TO MENTAL HEALTH JOURNALING

P icture yourself standing at the edge of a beautiful, unexplored landscape. Each path winds through different territories of thought and feeling, each clearing represents a new understanding waiting to unfold. This is your mental health landscape, rich with insights and possibilities for healing that will gradually reveal themselves through the practice of therapeutic journaling.

Just like a garden doesn't show you all its secrets at once, mental wellness unfolds naturally over time. Some insights bloom quickly, while others need gentle tending before they emerge. This journey isn't about forcing breakthroughs or racing to fix everything. It's about creating safe space for your authentic healing to emerge, one reflection at a time.

YOUR COMPANIONS ON THE PATH

I want you to get to know two fellow travelers who discovered healing through therapeutic writing. Sarah began journaling during a period when anxiety and perfectionism were over-whelming her daily life. At 34, she found herself caught in cycles of worry that affected her work, relationships, and sleep. Her mind constantly raced with what-if scenarios and harsh self-criticism that left her exhausted.

James started his practice at 42, seeking ways to navigate depression and isolation following a difficult divorce. He felt disconnected from friends and family, struggling with thoughts that convinced him he was a burden to others. Simple tasks felt overwhelming, and he questioned whether he'd ever feel like himself again.

Their stories show there's no single right way to explore your mental health through writing. Sarah's breakthrough came through recognizing thought patterns she'd never noticed before. James found healing in the simple act of putting his feelings into words, which helped them feel less frightening and more manageable.

"I thought therapeutic journaling meant writing deep insights about my problems," Sarah shares. "But some of my most meaningful discoveries came from messy, uncertain entries where I simply allowed myself to feel whatever was present. One morning, I just wrote 'I'm scared' over and over until tears appeared on the page. That moment of honesty opened up understanding I didn't know I needed."

James's experience revealed similar truths: "My first entries felt stilted, like I was writing a report about my symptoms. Then one evening, while describing a childhood memory, I found myself writing with raw emotion about experiences I thought I'd processed long ago. I realized therapeutic journaling isn't about analyzing my mental health. It's about befriending it."

SAFETY FIRST: UNDERSTANDING WHEN WRITING HELPS AND WHEN IT DOESN'T

Before we explore the tools and techniques ahead, you need to understand when therapeutic writing supports healing and when professional intervention is necessary. This knowledge protects your well-being and helps your writing practice serve your mental health rather than accidentally causing harm.

When Therapeutic Writing May Not Be Right for You:

Some situations require different approaches. If you have trouble identifying or describing emotions (called alexithymia), standard expressive writing approaches may feel frustrating rather than helpful. People experiencing hallucinations or delusions need professional supervision for any therapeutic work, including writing. If you've been through trauma in the past six months, please work with a trained trauma therapist rather than trying to process it alone through writing.

Warning Signs That Mean You Need Professional Support Right Away:

Stop writing and reach out for professional help if you experience ongoing distress lasting more than two hours after writing, increased rumination without any sense of processing or relief, compulsive writing that you cannot control or limit, or any worsening of your mental state that coincides with your writing practice. These signs suggest that writing may be accessing emotional material that needs professional support to process safely.

Crisis Resources to Keep Handy:

Keep these numbers easily accessible: National Suicide Prevention Lifeline (988), Crisis Text Line (text HOME to 741741), your local emergency services (911), and contact information for your current mental health providers if you have them. If you're currently in therapy, talk with your therapist about your therapeutic writing plans to make sure they work well together.

UNDERSTANDING YOUR EVIDENCE-BASED TOOLS

Think of the prompts in this book as different instruments in a complete mental health toolkit, each one designed for specific needs and backed by solid research on therapeutic writing effectiveness.

Daily Foundation Prompts work like gentle morning weather reports for your emotional landscape. These seven rotating prompts help you notice your inner climate with the same natural awareness you might check the day's weather. Studies show that brief, regular check-ins build emotional awareness more effectively than occasional intensive writing sessions.

Weekly Reflection Prompts reveal patterns in your mental health that daily entries might miss. These thirteen prompts help you step back and see connections across time. People who do weekly reviews get much better at identifying triggers, tracking progress, and adjusting coping strategies.

Monthly Deep Dives illuminate the larger seasons of your psychological landscape. These fifteen prompts invite exploration of core beliefs, long-term patterns, and deeper aspects of your mental health journey. Monthly reflection helps people integrate insights from shorter writing sessions and maintain long-term healing gains.

Situational Prompts serve as first-aid companions for specific mental health challenges. When anxiety strikes, when depression visits, when stress feels overwhelming, these sixty-five prompts offer targeted support based on evidence from cognitive behavioral therapy, mindfulness approaches, and trauma-informed care.

CREATING YOUR EVIDENCE-BASED PRACTICE

Your therapeutic writing practice should be as individual as you are, while incorporating the approaches that actually work best for mental health improvement. The science provides clear guidance on what helps most people heal.

Timing That Supports Healing:

Studies consistently show that 15 to 20-minute writing sessions provide the best therapeutic benefit. Shorter sessions don't allow enough time for emotional processing, while longer sessions can become overwhelming or counterproductive. Plan for three to four writing sessions per week rather than daily practice, which allows time for insights to settle between sessions.

Choose times when you naturally feel reflective and won't be interrupted. Many people find early morning works well because it sets a positive tone for the day and happens before stress builds up. Others prefer evening writing to process the day's experiences. Trust your natural rhythms while maintaining consistency in timing.

Space Requirements for Safe Processing:

Create a private, secure environment where you feel safe to explore difficult emotions without judgment. This might be a quiet corner of your home, a peaceful spot in nature, or anywhere you can write without interruption or observation. The key is psychological safety: knowing you won't be disturbed or judged.

Make sure you have crisis resources easily accessible in your writing space. Keep phone numbers for support services nearby and have a plan for reaching out if difficult emotions arise during writing sessions.

Tools: The Science of Handwriting vs. Digital:

Brain studies strongly favor handwriting over typing for therapeutic benefit. Brain scans show that handwriting activates broader neural networks than typing, engaging visual, motor, and cognitive regions simultaneously. This enhanced brain connectivity appears to be one way that writing creates therapeutic change.

Choose a journal that invites writing and a pen that flows easily. Many people find that special writing tools help create a sense of ritual and importance around their practice. However, don't let perfect tools become a barrier to starting. Any paper and pen will serve the therapeutic function.

Cultural and Individual Considerations:

Most therapeutic writing studies have included people from Western populations where individual emotional expression is culturally encouraged. If you come from a culture that emphasizes collective well-being over individual expression, you may need to adapt prompts to feel authentic and helpful.

Age also influences how people respond to therapeutic writing. Adolescents show smaller but still meaningful benefits compared to adults. Older adults may prefer reminiscence-based approaches over problem-focused writing. Trust your instincts about what feels right for your developmental stage and cultural background.

INTEGRATION WITH PROFESSIONAL TREATMENT

Therapeutic writing works best as a complement to professional mental health care rather than a replacement for it. If you're currently working with a therapist, psychiatrist, or other mental health provider, discuss your writing practice with them to make sure it supports your treatment goals.

Collaboration with Your Treatment Team:

Share relevant insights from your writing practice with your therapist during sessions. Many mental health professionals welcome therapeutic writing as homework between appointments. Your journal entries can provide valuable information about patterns, triggers, and progress that might not be apparent during brief therapy sessions.

If you're taking medication for mental health conditions, use writing to track your responses, side effects, and overall well-being. This information helps your prescribing provider make informed decisions about dosage and medication changes.

When Writing Complements Therapy:

Therapeutic writing can extend the benefits of therapy sessions by providing space to process insights between appointments. It can help you prepare for therapy sessions by clarifying what you want to discuss. Writing can also help you practice therapeutic techniques like cognitive restructuring or mindfulness between professional sessions.

Treatment Adherence and Goal Setting:

Use writing to explore your feelings about treatment, track your progress toward therapy goals, and maintain motivation during challenging periods. People who write about their treatment experiences show better adherence to therapy recommendations and medication regimens.

WHEN EMOTIONS INTENSIFY: KEEPING YOURSELF SAFE

Therapeutic writing often brings up strong emotions, which can be part of the healing process when handled properly. However, you need clear guidelines for managing emotional intensity safely.

Normal vs. Concerning Responses:

It's normal to feel some emotional intensity during therapeutic writing. You might experience sadness, anger, anxiety, or other difficult feelings as you explore mental health challenges. These responses typically fade within an hour or two of writing and often lead to a sense of relief or clarity.

Concerning responses include ongoing distress that doesn't diminish over several hours, increased symptoms of depression or anxiety that worsen after writing, or feeling overwhelmed by emotions that writing has brought up. These responses suggest you need professional support to process the material you're accessing.

Grounding Techniques for Emotional Regulation:

When emotions feel too intense during writing, stop and use grounding techniques to return to the present moment. Try the 5-4-3-2-1 technique: identify five things you can see, four things you can touch, three things you can hear, two things you can smell, and one thing you can taste.

Deep breathing can also help regulate your nervous system. Breathe in for four counts, hold for four counts, breathe out for six counts. Repeat until you feel more centered.

When to Pause or Stop:

Trust your instincts about when writing feels too intense. It's better to write for shorter periods regularly than to push through overwhelming emotions. You can always return to a prompt when you feel more resourced.

If a particular prompt consistently brings up intense reactions, consider working on that topic with a professional therapist rather than through self-guided writing.

SIGNS OF MENTAL HEALTH PROGRESS THROUGH WRITING

Progress in mental health often looks different than you might expect. Rather than measuring success by dramatic break-throughs or the absence of symptoms, notice the subtle shifts in how you relate to your mental health challenges.

Increased Emotional Awareness:

You might find yourself recognizing emotions more quickly and accurately. Instead of feeling "bad" or "stressed," you might notice specific feelings like disappointment, frustration, or worry. This emotional precision is a sign that your awareness is becoming more sophisticated.

Better Pattern Recognition:

Over time, you may start noticing connections between situa-tions, thoughts, feelings, and behaviors that you hadn't seen before. Perhaps you'll recognize that your anxiety increases on Sunday evenings, or that conflict with your partner typically follows particularly stressful work days.

Improved Emotional Regulation:

Progress might show up as shorter recovery times from difficult emotions, less intense reactions to triggers, or better ability to soothe yourself when distressed. You might notice you're less likely to get caught in rumination or catastrophic thinking.

Enhanced Self-Compassion:

One of the most important signs of progress is developing a kinder, more understanding relationship with yourself. You might notice less harsh self-criticism and more willingness to treat yourself with the same compassion you'd offer a good friend.

Sarah noticed her progress in unexpected ways: "It wasn't that my anxiety disappeared, but I started catching anxious thoughts earlier instead of letting them spiral. My journal helped me see that worry wasn't protecting me the way I thought it was. I developed this gentle voice that could talk back to anxiety instead of just believing everything it told me."

James found his progress in relationship changes: "I wasn't suddenly happy all the time, but I started reaching out to friends again instead of isolating. My writing helped me see that depression was telling me lies about being a burden. I could challenge those thoughts with evidence from my relationships instead of just accepting them as truth."

YOUR FIRST STEPS IN THERAPEUTIC WRITING

Beginning a therapeutic writing practice is like planting a garden for mental wellness, one seed at a time. Start small and trust that each entry, however brief, contributes to your healing and growth.

Week One: Establishing Safety and Rhythm

Choose one consistent time each day for a brief mental health check-in using the daily foundation prompts. Start with just 10 minutes of writing, focusing more on showing up consistently than on writing deep insights. Notice which times and places feel most natural for reflection.

Pay attention to your emotional responses during and after writing. This week is about learning how your system responds to therapeutic writing and establishing safety protocols that work for you.

Week Two: Deepening the Practice

Gradually increase your writing time to 15 to 20 minutes if that feels comfortable. When you have more time and space, try one of the weekly reflection prompts to begin noticing patterns across your daily entries.

Start to notice which prompts feel most accessible and which bring up more intense emotions. This information will help you pace your practice appropriately.

Building Long-Term Sustainability:

Remember what studies show: consistency matters more than intensity. Three to four writing sessions per week create more therapeutic benefit than daily writing that you can't sustain. Focus on building a rhythm that feels manageable and nourishing rather than burdensome.

James learned this lesson through experience: "I started trying to write every day for an hour, thinking more would be better. I burned out quickly and stopped writing altogether. When I returned to a gentler approach: 20 minutes three times a week, the practice became sustainable and much more helpful."

MOVING FORWARD WITH CONFIDENCE

Your journey into therapeutic writing begins with the understanding that healing happens gradually, in small moments of insight and self-compassion. The tools in this book are designed to support that process while keeping you safe along the way.

As Sarah reminds us: "Therapeutic writing isn't about fixing yourself or finding perfect answers. It's about developing a friendlier relationship with your own mental health. Each entry is like having a caring conversation with yourself, and that kindness builds up over time into real healing."

The daily foundation prompts await you in the next chapter, ready to help you begin this journey of mental wellness through writing. They're designed as gentle companions for your healing, offering different ways to check in with yourself and build the foundation for deeper therapeutic work.

Trust that you have everything you need to begin. Your willingness to explore your mental health with curiosity and compassion is the most important tool you bring to this practice. Everything else can be learned along the way.

TWO
DAILY FOUNDATION PROMPTS

L ike the first gentle light of dawn revealing a landscape, daily mental health check-ins illuminate the current state of your inner world. These foundation prompts serve as caring morning questions, inviting you to notice what stirs within as you begin each day with intention and awareness.

Think of these seven prompts as trusted companions on your healing journey. Each one opens a different window into understanding your mental health, offering fresh perspectives on your thoughts, feelings, and patterns. You might find yourself drawn to specific prompts more than others. Trust this natural attraction. It often signals where the most valuable insights await.

BEGINNING YOUR DAILY PRACTICE

Rather than cycling through all seven prompts each day, choose one that speaks to your current needs. Some mornings, you might feel called to explore your emotional landscape. Other days, you may need to examine stress patterns or reconnect with your inner strength. Let your intuition guide you toward the prompt that will serve your mental health best in this moment.

Brief, consistent mental health check-ins build emotional awareness more effectively than lengthy but sporadic writing sessions.
Aim for 10 to 15 minutes of focused reflection, creating a sustainable rhythm that supports your well-being without overwhelming your schedule.

DAILY FOUNDATION PROMPT 1: WHAT IS THE CURRENT WEATHER OF YOUR EMOTIONAL LANDSCAPE TODAY?

Emotions move through our inner world like weather patterns,
sometimes sunny and calm, other times stormy or unpredictable.
This prompt invites you to check in with your emotional climate
without judgment, simply noticing what's present in your
mental sky right now.

Sarah discovered how this simple question revealed hidden
patterns in her anxiety: "One morning, I noticed this familiar
cloudiness that I usually ignored while rushing to start my day.
Instead of pushing past it, I stayed with the feeling. Beneath the
surface fog, I found a deeper worry about a presentation that
was still three weeks away. This recognition helped me understand why I'd been feeling unsettled for days without knowing
why."

When working with this prompt, let yourself notice without
trying to change or fix anything. Your emotions aren't problems
to solve but messengers offering information about what matters
to you and what needs attention in your life.

Consider exploring: What's the dominant feeling tone as you
wake up? Where do you sense emotions in your body? How do
different feelings affect your energy and motivation? What
emotional weather patterns do you notice repeating over time?

James found this prompt particularly grounding during difficult
periods: "I started thinking of my depression like a weather
system rather than a personal failing. Some days brought heavy

clouds, others offered breaks of sunlight. This perspective helped me remember that weather always changes, even when you're in the middle of a storm."

DAILY FOUNDATION PROMPT 2: WHAT THOUGHTS ARE CREATING STRESS OR CALM IN YOUR MIND RIGHT NOW?

Your thoughts create the soundtrack of your mental health experience. Some thoughts generate anxiety and tension, while others bring peace and clarity. This prompt helps you tune into the mental chatter that shapes your emotional state and stress levels throughout the day.

Sarah found unexpected insight in tracking her thought patterns: "I noticed my mind constantly running commentary about my performance at work. Not just during important meetings, but while making coffee, checking email, even walking to my car. This background voice was exhausting me before my day even began. Recognizing this pattern was the first step toward changing it."

This isn't about judging your thoughts as good or bad, but about developing awareness of how different thinking patterns affect your mental health. Simply noticing thoughts reduces their automatic power over your emotions.

Explore questions like: What mental themes keep returning? Which thoughts speed up your heart rate or tighten your muscles? What thoughts naturally slow your breathing and relax your body? How do your thoughts change throughout the day?

James discovered how his thoughts amplified his depression: "I realized I was having thoughts about my thoughts. I'd feel sad, then criticize myself for feeling sad, then feel guilty about the criticism. Learning to observe this cycle without getting caught in it gave me space to respond differently."

DAILY FOUNDATION PROMPT 3: WHERE DO YOU FEEL TENSION OR EASE IN YOUR BODY TODAY?

Your body holds wisdom about your mental health that your mind might miss. Physical sensations often signal emotional states before you consciously recognize them. This prompt helps you develop body awareness that supports emotional regulation and stress management.

Strong connections exist between physical tension patterns and mental health symptoms. Learning to read your body's signals provides early warning systems for anxiety, depression, and stress while also revealing what genuinely supports your well-being.

Sarah noticed how her body communicated anxiety: "My shoulders carry my worry like invisible backpacks. When I started paying attention, I realized they'd tighten hours before I consciously noticed feeling anxious. This body awareness became like an early warning system that helped me use coping strategies before anxiety fully took hold."

As you work with this prompt, scan your body from head to toe, noticing areas of tightness, pain, or discomfort alongside places that feel relaxed and comfortable. Both types of sensation offer valuable information.

Consider exploring: Where does stress typically show up in your body? What physical sensations accompany different emotions? When does your body feel most at ease? How do different activities affect your physical comfort?

James found his body held memories of emotional experiences: "I noticed my chest would feel heavy even on days when my mood seemed okay. Paying attention to that sensation helped me recognize that I was processing grief about my divorce in layers, not all at once. My body was wiser about my healing timeline than my mind was."

DAILY FOUNDATION PROMPT 4: WHAT SMALL ACT OF SELF-CARE DOES YOUR MENTAL HEALTH NEED TODAY?

Self-care isn't luxury. It's practical mental health maintenance. This prompt helps you tune into what would genuinely support your well-being today, moving beyond generic advice to discover what your specific mental health needs in this moment.

Effective self-care varies from person to person and day to day. Sometimes your mental health needs movement, other times rest. You might need connection or solitude, structure or flexibility, stimulation or calm. Learning to read these needs accurately improves your ability to support your own mental wellness.

Sarah learned to distinguish between surface wants and deeper needs: "I thought self-care meant bubble baths and shopping, but those never made me feel better. When I started really listening, I realized my mental health often needed me to say no to social plans when I was overwhelmed, or to have real conversations instead of small talk when I felt disconnected."

This prompt works best when you approach it with genuine curiosity rather than predetermined ideas about what self-care should look like. Trust your instincts about what would feel nourishing rather than what you think you should do.

Explore questions like: What would help you feel more grounded today? What type of energy do you need, calming or energizing? Do you need more connection or more solitude? What boundaries would support your well-being today?

James discovered that self-care could be surprisingly simple: "Sometimes my mental health just needed me to eat regular meals or go to bed on time. During depressive episodes, basic care felt like radical acts of kindness toward myself. The small things often made bigger differences than elaborate self-care routines."

DAILY FOUNDATION PROMPT 5: WHAT WORRY WANTS TO BE ACKNOWLEDGED AND THEN RELEASED?

Worry often persists because it feels unheard. This prompt creates space to acknowledge anxious thoughts without letting them dominate your mental landscape. Writing about worries can reduce their intensity and frequency.

The key is acknowledging worry without feeding it. Give your anxious thoughts a few minutes of attention, then consciously choose to release them rather than carrying them throughout your day. This practice helps prevent worry from building into overwhelming anxiety.

Sarah found this prompt helped break her rumination cycles: "Instead of trying to solve every worry or push anxious thoughts away, I started treating them like visitors who needed to be heard but didn't need to stay for dinner. Acknowledging my worries for a few minutes often satisfied whatever part of me generated them."

When working with this prompt, write down your worry clearly, explore what it's trying to protect you from, then consciously choose to set it aside. You can always return to legitimate concerns during appropriate problem-solving time.

Consider: What specific worries are cycling through your mind? What is this worry trying to protect you from? Which concerns deserve action and which need to be released? How can you honor anxious thoughts without letting them control your day?

James learned to distinguish between productive concern and anxious rumination: "I realized most of my worries were about things I couldn't control or problems that didn't actually exist yet. Writing them down helped me see which ones deserved attention and which ones were just my mind spinning stories about imaginary futures."

DAILY FOUNDATION PROMPT 6: WHAT STRENGTH OR RESILIENCE ARE YOU NOTICING IN YOURSELF TODAY?

Mental health challenges can overshadow your natural resilience and capabilities. This prompt helps you recognize the strength you're already demonstrating, even during difficult periods. Building awareness of your resilience improves self-confidence and emotional regulation.

People who regularly acknowledge their strengths show better mental health outcomes and greater recovery from setbacks. This isn't about forced positivity but about accurate recognition of your actual capabilities and resources.

Sarah discovered strength in unexpected places: "I was so focused on my anxiety symptoms that I missed all the ways I was coping effectively. When I started looking for resilience, I realized I was showing up for friends, meeting work deadlines, and taking care of my health even while struggling. That was actually pretty remarkable."

Look for strength in small actions as well as major accomplishments. Getting out of bed during depression demonstrates resilience. Managing anxiety while completing necessary tasks shows courage. Asking for help when you need it reveals wisdom.

Explore questions like: What challenges are you navigating right now? How are you taking care of yourself or others? What positive choices are you making despite difficulties? Where do you see growth or learning happening?

James found this prompt shifted his relationship with depression: "Instead of seeing depression as pure weakness, I started noticing the strength it took to keep functioning when everything felt heavy. I was still showing up for my students, still calling my mom, still feeding myself. Depression wasn't erasing my resilience. It was making it more visible."

DAILY FOUNDATION PROMPT 7: WHAT INTENTION CAN GUIDE YOUR MENTAL WELLNESS TODAY?

Intentions differ from goals by focusing on how you want to be rather than what you want to achieve. This prompt helps you set a gentle direction for your mental health that can guide decisions throughout your day without creating pressure or stress.

Effective mental health intentions are specific enough to provide guidance but flexible enough to adapt to changing circumstances. They might focus on emotional regulation, relationship quality, self-compassion, or any aspect of well-being that needs attention.

Sarah learned to set intentions that supported rather than stressed her: "I used to set goals like 'don't be anxious today,' which just made me anxious about being anxious. When I switched to intentions like 'notice anxiety with kindness' or 'choose calm responses when possible,' I had something helpful to return to instead of impossible standards to meet."

Your intention might be as simple as "breathe deeply when stressed" or "speak to myself with compassion." The power lies not in perfect execution but in having a touchstone that guides you back to mental wellness throughout your day.

Consider: How do you want to relate to difficult emotions today? What quality do you want to bring to your interactions? How do you want to treat yourself when challenges arise? What would support your mental health best today?

James found intentions more sustainable than rigid mental health rules: "My intention might be 'reach out instead of isolating' or 'trust that this feeling will pass.' These gave me direction without demanding perfection. When I struggled, I could return to my intention instead of judging myself for not following complicated mental health protocols."

WORKING WITH THESE PROMPTS OVER TIME

Like tending a garden through changing seasons, your relationship with these prompts will evolve naturally. Some prompts might feel immediately accessible, while others require patience before revealing their insights. This evolution is natural and valuable, showing different aspects of yourself as you grow.

Sarah discovered how her practice deepened: "At first, I tried to use every prompt every day, treating them like tasks to complete. This left me feeling scattered. When I learned to listen for which prompt called to me each morning, my practice became much more meaningful. Some weeks I stayed with the same prompt for days, discovering new layers each time."

James found value in reviewing his daily entries weekly: "Looking back over several days of writing helped me notice patterns I couldn't see in individual moments. My relationship with stress showed up differently through different prompts, but themes emerged when I stepped back and looked at the bigger picture."

Guidelines for Sustainable Practice:

Stay curious about how different prompts resonate at different times. Your natural attraction or resistance to certain prompts often carries valuable information about what's ready to be explored.

Allow your responses to vary in length and depth. Some days might bring flowing insights, others just a few honest observations. Both serve your mental health journey.

Notice how insights build upon each other. An observation about emotions today might illuminate a stress pattern you recognize next week, which could reveal a self-care need you hadn't considered before.

Trust that understanding develops gradually. Some insights need time to unfold before revealing their full meaning. Others might shift and evolve as your mental health changes.

MOVING INTO WEEKLY REFLECTION

As you develop comfort with daily mental health check-ins, you might notice larger patterns and themes emerging in your awareness. This natural evolution leads us toward weekly reflection, which helps you recognize the broader rhythms of your mental wellness.

Think of daily prompts as gathering individual moments of self-awareness. Weekly reflection allows you to step back and notice the streams and currents they form when viewed together. These wider perspectives reveal how individual moments connect into meaningful patterns that can guide your mental health care.

Sarah describes this progression: "Daily prompts helped me develop regular mental health awareness. When I began working with weekly reflections, I discovered how these daily insights wove together into larger understanding. Patterns I couldn't see day by day became clear when viewed through a wider lens."

The foundation you're building through daily practice creates the perfect groundwork for the deeper exploration waiting in weekly reflection. Your growing ability to notice thoughts, feelings, and patterns will serve as powerful tools for understanding the bigger picture of your mental health journey.

Trust the wisdom you've developed through consistent practice as we explore these broader perspectives together. Your daily awareness becomes the foundation for recognizing the larger rhythms and patterns that shape your emotional well-being.

THREE
WEEKLY REFLECTION
PROMPTS

I magine walking a familiar path each day, noticing individual moments, changes in your mental landscape, and small shifts in your emotional weather. Then, once a week, you climb to a gentle overlook that reveals how these daily observations connect into larger patterns. This is the relationship between daily mental health check-ins and weekly reflection.

Weekly reflection doesn't replace your daily practice. Instead, it offers a wider lens through which to view your mental health journey. Think of daily prompts as gathering precious insights, while weekly reflection helps you arrange them into meaningful patterns that can guide your healing and growth.

CREATING SPACE FOR WEEKLY MENTAL HEALTH PRACTICE

Sarah discovered the natural rhythm of combining daily and weekly reflection: "I protect my morning journaling time like a sacred ritual. Those quiet moments with coffee and my journal anchor my days and help me notice what's happening in my mental health. But Sunday evenings have become equally important. A special time when I curl up in my favorite chair, review my daily entries, and let myself see the larger stories emerging from my week."

James found his weekly rhythm differently: "Friday afternoons work best for me. After the week settles, I take my journal to a quiet coffee shop. Having that physical separation helps me step back and see patterns I miss when I'm in the middle of daily experiences. I still write every morning, but this weekly pause helps me understand how my daily insights connect to bigger themes in my mental health."

THE INTEGRATION OF DAILY AND WEEKLY PRACTICE

Your daily mental health writing builds a foundation of self-awareness, capturing moments, feelings, and observations as they arise. Weekly reflection then invites you to notice how these pieces fit together into patterns that can inform your mental health care.

Guidelines for Effective Integration:

Keep your daily writing spontaneous and authentic. Let each morning's reflection flow naturally without worrying about weekly themes or patterns that might emerge later.

Choose a weekly time that feels spacious and nurturing. Whether it's Sunday morning with tea, Friday afternoon in nature, or Saturday evening by candlelight, make this time different from your daily practice.

Begin your weekly reflection by gently reviewing your daily entries. Notice what stands out, what patterns emerge, and what themes seem to be asking for attention.

Trust that some weekly reflections will feel deeper than others. Like daily journaling, this practice has its own natural rhythm of insight and integration.

WEEKLY REFLECTION PROMPT 1: WHAT PATTERNS IN YOUR ANXIETY OR STRESS DID YOU NOTICE THIS WEEK?

Anxiety and stress often speak in whispers before they shout. A feeling that returns in certain situations, a physical tension that appears with specific people, or a worry that keeps nudging at your awareness. This prompt invites you to notice these gentle repetitions and explore what they might be trying to communicate about your mental health needs.

Sarah discovered an unexpected pattern during her weekly reflection: "Looking through my daily entries, I noticed how often I mentioned feeling 'just a little on edge' before family phone calls. At first, this seemed like normal nervousness. But sitting with this pattern revealed something deeper. The edginess appeared most consistently before conversations where I felt pressure to have my life figured out. This recognition helped me understand why family support sometimes felt stressful instead of comforting."

When exploring patterns in your anxiety and stress, consider situations that repeatedly stirred tension, thoughts that consistently increased your worry, physical sensations that appeared in similar circumstances, and times when stress felt manageable versus overwhelming.

James found his stress patterns through weekly review: "Reading through my entries, I realized my worst anxiety days followed nights when I stayed up late scrolling on my phone. It wasn't just about being tired. The combination of sleep deprivation and digital overstimulation was priming my nervous system for anxiety the next day. Understanding this connection helped me set boundaries that actually supported my mental health."

Remember that patterns aren't problems to solve immediately. They're more like weather systems in your mental health landscape, each one offering information about what supports or stresses your well-being. Some patterns might invite change, while others simply need to be understood with compassion.

WEEKLY REFLECTION PROMPT 2: HOW DID YOUR COPING STRATEGIES SERVE YOU THIS WEEK?

Your coping strategies are the tools you use to navigate mental health challenges, from formal techniques learned in therapy to informal habits you've developed over time. This prompt helps you evaluate which strategies genuinely support your well-being and which might need adjustment or replacement.

People often continue using coping strategies that once helped but no longer serve their current needs. Weekly reflection provides space to honestly assess what's working and what isn't, allowing you to refine your mental health toolkit.

Sarah discovered both helpful and unhelpful coping patterns: "I realized I was still using distraction techniques that worked during college but weren't serving my adult anxiety. Binge-watching shows helped me avoid immediate stress but left me feeling worse the next day. When I paid attention to the aftermath of different coping strategies, I could make better choices about which ones actually helped my mental health."

As you explore this prompt, notice which strategies genuinely calmed your nervous system versus those that just postponed difficult feelings. Consider what helps you feel more resourced and capable versus what leaves you feeling depleted or disconnected.

Examine both formal coping skills like breathing exercises or mindfulness techniques, and informal strategies like calling friends, taking walks, or engaging in creative activities. All forms of coping deserve honest evaluation.

James found that some of his coping strategies were actually maintaining his depression: "I thought staying busy was helping me manage sadness, but weekly reflection showed me that constant activity was preventing me from processing my emotions. When I allowed myself quiet time to feel what I was feeling, my mood actually improved instead of getting worse."

WEEKLY REFLECTION PROMPT 3: WHAT TRIGGERED YOUR STRONGEST EMOTIONAL REACTIONS THIS WEEK?

Understanding your emotional triggers provides valuable information about what matters deeply to you, what old wounds might need healing, and what current situations require different approaches. This prompt helps you develop emotional intelligence by examining what consistently activates intense responses.

Triggers aren't character flaws or signs of weakness. They're information about where your nervous system feels threatened or where past experiences continue to influence present reactions. Approaching triggers with curiosity rather than judgment creates space for healing and growth.

Sarah found unexpected insights in examining her triggers: "I noticed that my strongest reactions happened when people questioned my decisions, even in casual conversation. This wasn't about the specific topics but about feeling like I had to justify my choices. Understanding this trigger helped me see how much energy I spent defending myself instead of simply living my life."

When working with this prompt, notice both obvious triggers that create immediate intense reactions and subtler ones that gradually build emotional charge over time. Consider what themes connect different triggering situations and what these reactions might be trying to protect or communicate.

James discovered layers in his emotional triggers: "My biggest reactions seemed random until I looked for patterns. They all involved feeling unseen or misunderstood. Once I recognized this theme, I could communicate my needs more clearly instead of just reacting defensively when it happened."

Remember that identifying triggers is the first step toward healing them, not eliminating all situations that might activate them. The goal is developing the emotional regulation skills to respond rather than react when triggers arise.

WEEKLY REFLECTION PROMPT 4: WHERE DID YOU SHOW YOURSELF COMPASSION THIS WEEK?

Self-compassion is one of the most powerful tools for mental health recovery and maintenance, yet many people struggle to recognize when they're already practicing it. This prompt helps you notice acts of kindness toward yourself, building awareness that can strengthen this crucial mental health skill.

Self-compassion improves emotional regulation, reduces anxiety and depression, and increases resilience. People who treat themselves with kindness recover more quickly from setbacks and maintain better mental health over time.

Sarah learned to recognize subtle forms of self-compassion: "I was looking for grand gestures of self-care but missing all the small ways I was already being kind to myself. Choosing not to check work email after dinner, letting myself rest when I felt tired, speaking up when I needed help. These weren't dramatic acts but they were authentic expressions of self-care."

Self-compassion often appears in moments when you choose understanding over self-criticism, when you meet your own needs without guilt, when you forgive yourself for mistakes, or when you treat yourself with the same kindness you'd offer a good friend.

Notice both planned acts of self-compassion and spontaneous moments when you naturally treated yourself well. Consider what made these moments possible and what barriers typically interfere with self-kindness.

James found that self-compassion could be surprisingly practical: "I expected self-compassion to feel warm and fuzzy, but often it was just practical kindness. Like not pushing myself to socialize when I needed quiet time, or eating regular meals during depressive episodes. Self-compassion turned out to be about honoring my actual needs instead of judging them."

WEEKLY REFLECTION PROMPT 5: WHAT NEGATIVE THOUGHT PATTERNS KEPT RECURRING THIS WEEK?

Negative thought patterns are like well-worn paths in your mental landscape. Easy to follow but not always leading where you want to go. This prompt helps you identify repetitive thoughts that contribute to anxiety, depression, or other mental health challenges, creating awareness that's the first step toward change.

Simply noticing negative thought patterns reduces their automatic power over your emotions. You don't need to eliminate negative thoughts entirely, but developing awareness helps you choose whether to follow or redirect them.

Sarah discovered how her thought patterns maintained her anxiety: "I realized I was constantly running worst-case scenario planning in my head. For every situation, my mind would immediately jump to what could go wrong and how I should prepare for disaster. This mental habit was exhausting me and preventing me from enjoying anything good that was actually happening."

Common negative thought patterns include catastrophizing, all-or-nothing thinking, mind reading, fortune telling, and personalizing situations that aren't actually about you. Notice which patterns appear most frequently in your mental health experience.

Examine both obvious negative thoughts and subtler patterns that might seem helpful but actually increase distress. Sometimes thoughts that appear protective or productive are actually maintaining mental health symptoms.

James recognized how his thought patterns fed his depression: "I was constantly comparing my internal experience to other people's external appearances, deciding I was failing at life because everyone else seemed to have it together. This comparison habit was making my depression worse by convincing me that feeling sad meant something was fundamentally wrong with me."

WEEKLY REFLECTION PROMPT 6: HOW DID CONNECTION WITH OTHERS IMPACT YOUR MENTAL HEALTH THIS WEEK?

Human beings are wired for connection, and your relationships significantly influence your mental health. This prompt helps you understand how different types of social interaction affect your well-being, guiding you toward connections that support your healing and growth.

Social support is one of the strongest predictors of mental health resilience. However, not all social interaction provides equal benefit. Some relationships energize and restore you, while others might drain your resources or trigger difficult emotions.

Sarah learned to distinguish between different types of social interaction: "I assumed all socializing was good for my mental health, but weekly reflection showed me that surface-level social activities often left me feeling more isolated than before. The connections that genuinely helped my anxiety were ones where I could be authentic rather than performing happiness."

Consider both formal social support from friends and family and informal connections with colleagues, neighbors, or acquaintances. Notice which interactions left you feeling more connected to yourself and others versus those that felt draining or inauthentic.

Examine how isolation versus connection affected your mood, energy, and overall mental health. Some people recharge through solitude while others need regular social contact to maintain emotional balance.

James found unexpected patterns in his social needs: "During my depression, I thought I needed constant social stimulation to feel better. But weekly reflection showed me that quiet, one-on-one conversations were much more healing than group activities. Large social gatherings actually increased my sense of isolation because I felt like I had to pretend to be okay."

WEEKLY REFLECTION PROMPT 7: WHAT MOMENTS BROUGHT YOU GENUINE PEACE OR JOY THIS WEEK?

Mental health challenges can overshadow moments of genuine well-being, making it harder to recognize what naturally supports your emotional balance. This prompt helps you identify experiences that bring authentic peace or joy, building awareness of what nourishes your mental health.

People who regularly notice positive experiences maintain better mental health and recover more quickly from difficult periods. This isn't about forced positivity but about accurate recognition of what genuinely feels good.

Sarah discovered joy in unexpected places: "The moments that brought me real peace weren't the ones I planned for happiness. They were small, unscripted times: watching my neighbor's cat sunbathe, having a genuine laugh with a coworker, feeling completely absorbed while cooking dinner. These moments felt true in a way that forced fun activities never did."

Look for both obvious sources of joy and subtle moments of contentment or peace. Consider what made these experiences possible and what they might tell you about what your mental health needs to thrive.

Notice whether positive moments happened during solitude or connection, activity or rest, routine or novelty. These patterns provide valuable information about what conditions support your well-being.

James recognized that joy often appeared when he stopped trying to manufacture it: "My best moments happened when I wasn't monitoring my mood or trying to feel better. Playing guitar without worrying about getting better at it, having coffee without checking my phone, walking without destination or timeline. Joy seemed to find me more easily when I relaxed my grip on needing to feel happy."

WEEKLY REFLECTION PROMPT 8: HOW DID YOUR SLEEP, EXERCISE, AND NUTRITION AFFECT YOUR MENTAL STATE THIS WEEK?

Your physical health provides the foundation for your mental health. Sleep, movement, and nutrition directly influence mood regulation, stress resilience, and cognitive function. This prompt helps you understand how lifestyle factors impact your emotional well-being.

Strong connections exist between physical and mental health. Sleep deprivation makes anxiety and depression worse. Regular movement improves mood regulation. Stable blood sugar supports emotional stability. However, the specific relationships vary from person to person.

Sarah learned to track these connections without judgment: "I realized that skipping meals didn't just make me hungry. It made me anxious and irritable. When I noticed this pattern, I could address my physical needs before they triggered mental health symptoms. It wasn't about perfect nutrition but about understanding how my body's needs affected my emotional state."

Notice how different sleep patterns influenced your mood, energy, and stress levels. Consider what types of movement or physical activity supported your mental health versus what felt overwhelming or unhelpful.

Examine how eating patterns, meal timing, and food choices affected your emotional regulation and overall well-being. Look for connections without creating rigid rules about what you should or shouldn't do.

James found that small physical changes created significant mental health improvements: "I discovered that taking short walks during my lunch break had a bigger impact on my depression than hour-long gym sessions that I rarely maintained. Understanding what physical activities actually felt sustainable helped me create lifestyle changes that supported rather than stressed my mental health."

WEEKLY REFLECTION PROMPT 9: WHAT BOUNDARIES SERVED YOUR MENTAL HEALTH THIS WEEK?

Boundaries are practical tools for protecting your mental health, not walls that isolate you from others. This prompt helps you recognize when setting limits supported your well-being and when unclear boundaries might have contributed to stress or overwhelm.

Healthy boundaries look different for everyone and vary based on current mental health needs. Sometimes you need boundaries around time, energy, or emotional availability. Other times you might need limits on topics of conversation, types of activities, or social commitments.

Sarah discovered that boundaries could be surprisingly gentle: "I always thought boundaries meant having difficult conversations or disappointing people. But this week I noticed how saying 'let me check my calendar and get back to you' instead of immediately saying yes gave me space to consider what I actually had capacity for. Small boundaries were often more effective than dramatic ones."

Consider boundaries you set around your time, energy, emotional availability, or personal space. Notice which boundaries felt easy to maintain and which required more effort or caused anxiety.

Examine situations where you wish you had set clearer boundaries and times when boundaries you set genuinely supported your mental health. Both types of experiences provide valuable learning.

James learned that boundaries were acts of self-respect: "I realized that when I didn't set boundaries, I ended up resenting people for things they didn't even know they were doing. Setting clear limits actually improved my relationships because I could show up more authentically when I wasn't feeling overwhelmed or taken advantage of."

WEEKLY REFLECTION PROMPT 10: WHERE DID YOU PRACTICE MINDFULNESS OR PRESENT-MOMENT AWARENESS THIS WEEK?

Mindfulness, the practice of paying attention to the present moment without judgment, is one of the most studied tools for mental health improvement. This prompt helps you notice when you naturally accessed present-moment awareness and how it affected your well-being.

You don't need formal meditation practice to experience mindfulness. Present-moment awareness can happen while eating, walking, listening to music, or having conversations. The key is noticing when your attention rests fully in your current experience rather than being caught in thoughts about the past or future.

Sarah found mindfulness in everyday activities: "I noticed that washing dishes mindfully, actually feeling the warm water and focusing on the simple task, calmed my anxiety more than trying to meditate when I was already agitated. Mindfulness worked best for me when it was integrated into normal activities rather than being a separate practice I had to remember to do."

Consider moments when you felt fully present and engaged with your current experience. Notice what activities naturally draw your attention into the present moment and how this awareness affects your mental state.

Examine both formal mindfulness practices and informal moments of present-moment awareness. Both contribute to mental health improvement through increased emotional regulation and reduced rumination.

James discovered that mindfulness helped him relate differently to difficult emotions: "Instead of trying to push away sad feelings or analyze them endlessly, I started just noticing them with curiosity. This present-moment awareness didn't make depression disappear, but it helped me stop fighting it so hard, which actually made it more manageable."

WEEKLY REFLECTION PROMPT 11: WHAT CHALLENGED YOUR RESILIENCE THIS WEEK, AND HOW DID YOU RESPOND?

Resilience isn't the absence of difficulty but your capacity to navigate challenges while maintaining your mental health and sense of self. This prompt helps you recognize both what tests your resilience and how you're already demonstrating strength in difficult situations.

Building resilience awareness helps you understand your own coping capacity and develop confidence in your ability to handle future challenges. It also reveals which strategies genuinely support you during tough times versus which ones might need adjustment.

Sarah learned to recognize resilience in small responses: "I was looking for dramatic examples of overcoming adversity but missing all the ways I was showing resilience every day. Managing work stress while dealing with family problems, maintaining friendships during my own difficult period, getting up each morning despite feeling anxious. These were all demonstrations of strength I hadn't acknowledged."

Consider both major challenges that tested your limits and smaller daily stressors that required resilience. Notice how you responded in moments of difficulty and what resources you drew upon to navigate them.

Examine what helped you bounce back from setbacks and what made challenges feel more overwhelming. This information helps you understand what supports your resilience versus what depletes it.

James found that resilience often looked different than he expected: "I thought resilience meant pushing through everything without feeling affected. But this week I realized that asking for help when I needed it, taking breaks when I felt overwhelmed, and admitting when things were hard were actually signs of strength, not weakness."

WEEKLY REFLECTION PROMPT 12: HOW DID YOUR RELATIONSHIP WITH YOURSELF EVOLVE THIS WEEK?

Your relationship with yourself, how you talk to yourself, treat your needs, and respond to your own struggles, significantly influences your mental health. This prompt helps you notice shifts in self-compassion, self-acceptance, and overall self-relationship.

Many people are harder on themselves than they would ever be on a friend. Developing a kinder, more understanding relationship with yourself improves emotional regulation, reduces anxiety and depression, and supports overall mental wellness.

Sarah noticed subtle changes in her internal dialogue: "I realized I was starting to catch myself when my inner critic got really harsh, not to stop the thoughts completely but to question whether they were actually helpful. Instead of believing every critical thought, I started asking whether I would talk to a friend the way I was talking to myself."

Consider how you spoke to yourself during difficult moments, how you responded to your own mistakes or struggles, what needs you honored or ignored, and how your self-compassion showed up or was absent.

Notice changes in how you relate to your mental health symptoms, your personal needs, and your growth process. Both improvements and setbacks in self-relationship provide valuable information.

James found that his self-relationship evolved gradually: "I didn't suddenly start loving myself or anything dramatic like that. But I noticed I was becoming less mean to myself when I felt depressed. Instead of criticizing myself for feeling sad, I started treating depression more like a weather system that required appropriate care rather than judgment."

WEEKLY REFLECTION PROMPT 13: WHAT PROGRESS IN YOUR MENTAL HEALTH JOURNEY CAN YOU ACKNOWLEDGE THIS WEEK?

Progress in mental health often appears in subtle forms that are easy to miss if you're only looking for dramatic improvements. This prompt helps you recognize real advances in your emotional well-being, coping skills, and overall mental health management.

Mental health progress might look like shorter recovery times from difficult emotions, better recognition of your own patterns, increased willingness to seek support, or improved ability to distinguish between thoughts and reality. Small advances build up over time into meaningful change.

Sarah learned to appreciate gradual progress: "I expected mental health progress to feel like switches being flipped, from anxious to calm, from struggling to thriving. Instead, progress looked like noticing my anxiety earlier, having kinder responses to myself when I struggled, and gradually feeling less afraid of my own emotions."

Consider improvements in emotional awareness, coping strategies, relationship skills, or self-compassion. Notice increased resilience, better boundary setting, or enhanced ability to ask for what you need.

Examine both obvious advances and subtle shifts that might be easy to overlook. Sometimes the most important progress happens in how you relate to challenges rather than in the absence of difficulties.

James recognized progress in unexpected areas: "My depression symptoms weren't completely gone, but I was handling them differently. I could feel sad without panicking about feeling sad. I could have low energy days without deciding I was failing at life. Progress looked like making friends with my own mental health instead of fighting it constantly."

BUILDING YOUR WEEKLY PRACTICE

Your weekly mental health reflection practice is like tending a garden that reveals different treasures as you spend consistent time with it. It's not about forcing insights or checking prompts off a list but about creating gentle space for understanding to emerge naturally.

Creating Sustainable Rhythm:

Choose a consistent time each week that feels spacious and peaceful. This might be Sunday morning with coffee, Friday evening as the week winds down, or any time when you can reflect without rushing.

Begin by reading through your daily entries from the week, not to judge or analyze but simply to notice what patterns or themes catch your attention. Trust that the insights that need your awareness will naturally stand out.

Use the weekly prompts as guides rather than assignments. Some weeks, one prompt might provide rich exploration. Other weeks, you might touch on several different themes. Let your current needs and interests guide your focus.

When Weekly Reflection Feels Difficult:

Some weeks bring insights easily, while others might feel unclear or emotionally challenging. Both experiences serve your mental health growth. If reflection feels overwhelming, focus on just one small pattern or moment from the week rather than trying to analyze everything.

Remember that weekly reflection is meant to support, not stress, your mental health. If a particular week's exploration brings up intense emotions, consider sharing those insights with a therapist or trusted friend rather than processing them alone.

MOVING TOWARD DEEPER UNDERSTANDING

As you develop comfort with daily check-ins and weekly pattern recognition, you might notice even larger themes and cycles emerging in your mental health journey. This natural progression leads us toward monthly reflection, which helps you understand the seasonal rhythms of your emotional landscape.

Monthly reflection doesn't replace your daily or weekly practice. Instead, it adds another layer of insight, helping you see how weeks connect into months and how longer-term patterns shape your mental health experience.

Sarah reflects on this evolution: "Daily writing helped me notice what was happening moment to moment. Weekly reflection showed me patterns I couldn't see day by day. But something in me felt ready for an even wider view, for understanding the deeper currents that shape my choices and relationships over longer periods."

Your growing ability to notice patterns and sit with uncertainty through daily and weekly practice creates a strong foundation for deeper exploration. Like developing emotional muscle, your capacity for self-understanding grows naturally as you create space for different rhythms of reflection.

As we prepare to explore monthly deep dives together, carry with you the trust you've developed in your own way of understanding. Remember that each way of reflecting serves its own purpose in your mental health journey.

FOUR
MONTHLY DEEP DIVES

ave you ever stepped back from a garden to see its true
patterns? Maybe you've walked through a landscape
daily, noticing individual flowers and changes, then climbed a
hill and suddenly seen how all the different sections work
together as a living whole. This is your mental health landscape,
rich with insights and possibilities for healing that reveal themselves through the practice of monthly reflection.

Think of it this way: daily reflection helps you notice individual
thoughts and feelings, weekly reflection shows you how
different patterns interact, and monthly reflection lets you see
the whole ecosystem of your mental health changing through
longer cycles. Here, you begin to recognize the seasonal rhythms
that shape your emotional well-being and psychological growth.

DISCOVERING YOUR MENTAL HEALTH LANDSCAPE

Sarah discovered this wider perspective quite naturally: "I used
to think monthly reflection meant analyzing everything that
happened in the past four weeks, which felt overwhelming. But
one quiet Sunday afternoon, I spread out all my journal entries

on my living room floor, made some tea, and just let myself notice what themes caught my attention. Things that seemed random in the moment started appearing like threads in a tapestry. I realized how often my anxiety spikes connected to upcoming changes, even positive ones. This wasn't about judging myself but finally seeing a pattern that had been invisible when I was too close to it."

James found his monthly practice evolved with patience: "At first, monthly reflection felt like too much emotional territory to cover. Then I started treating it more like visiting with an old friend who knows me well. I'd take my journal to this peaceful park I love, find a comfortable bench, and just spend time with my own story. Sometimes I notice practical things, like how my energy cycles through the month. Other times, I discover deeper patterns, like how my need for control shows up in different disguises when I'm stressed."

Monthly reflection isn't about analyzing everything or finding things to fix. It's more like giving yourself the gift of perspective. Imagine sitting with a wise therapist who knows your history well, looking back over your journey with understanding and compassion. This kind of reflection helps you recognize the larger stories playing out in your mental health, the deeper currents that influence your emotional responses and relationship patterns.

MONTHLY DEEP DIVE PROMPT 1: WHAT CORE BELIEFS ABOUT YOURSELF HAVE BEEN CHALLENGED OR CONFIRMED THIS MONTH?

Core beliefs are the basic assumptions you hold about yourself, others, and the world. They often operate beneath conscious awareness but significantly influence your mental health, emotional responses, and life choices. This month, let's gently explore which beliefs might be shifting or becoming more solid through your experiences.

Sarah noticed a surprising shift: "Looking back through a month of entries, something interesting emerged. I've always believed I was basically selfish because I need alone time and can't handle constant social interaction. But this month, several friends specifically thanked me for being there during their difficult times. I started wondering if taking care of my own needs actually made me more available for others, not less. This wasn't a dramatic revelation but a quiet questioning of an old story I'd been carrying."

Core beliefs often reveal themselves through your emotional reactions, the patterns you notice repeating, and the internal stories that arise during challenges. They might be beliefs about your worthiness, capability, lovability, or place in the world.

When working with this prompt, notice which beliefs felt shaken by new experiences and which felt strengthened by evidence. Consider beliefs that served you well in the past but might be ready for updating, and assumptions about yourself that recent experiences have either challenged or confirmed.

James discovered his beliefs shifting gradually: "I realized I'd been operating under the assumption that needing help meant I was weak or failing somehow. But this month, when I asked my neighbor for assistance moving furniture and he seemed genuinely happy to help, it challenged this belief. Maybe interdependence was normal rather than a sign of inadequacy. This shift didn't happen overnight, but I could see it beginning in my journal entries."

Remember that challenging core beliefs can feel unsettling because they've provided stability, even when they weren't entirely accurate or helpful. Be patient with yourself as old assumptions shift and new understandings emerge.

MONTHLY DEEP DIVE PROMPT 2: HOW HAS YOUR RELATIONSHIP WITH ANXIETY, DEPRESSION, OR OTHER MENTAL HEALTH CHALLENGES EVOLVED THIS MONTH?

Your relationship with mental health symptoms, how you relate to, understand, and respond to them, often matters as much as the symptoms themselves. This prompt invites exploration of whether that relationship has shifted, deepened, or changed in any way during the past month.

Many people begin their mental health journey seeing symptoms as enemies to defeat rather than experiences to understand. Over time, some discover that fighting their mental health creates additional suffering, while accepting and working with symptoms can reduce their intensity and impact.

Sarah found her relationship with anxiety evolving: "I noticed something different in how I related to anxious feelings this month. Instead of immediately trying to make anxiety go away or criticizing myself for feeling worried, I started getting curious about what my anxiety was trying to protect me from. This didn't eliminate anxious feelings, but it made them feel less frightening and more like information I could use."

Consider how you've been speaking to yourself about your mental health challenges, what strategies you've used to cope with difficult symptoms, how your understanding of your conditions has shifted, and whether your tolerance for difficult emotions has changed.

Notice both improvements in your relationship with mental health and times when old patterns of self-criticism or avoidance returned. Both directions of movement provide valuable information about your healing process.

James discovered a gentler approach to depression: "This month, instead of treating my low energy days like personal failures, I started thinking of them more like weather systems that required appropriate responses. Some days called for indoor activities and rest, just like rainy days call for different choices than sunny ones. This perspective didn't cure my depression, but it reduced the shame and self-criticism that used to make difficult days even harder."

MONTHLY DEEP DIVE PROMPT 3: WHAT PATTERNS IN YOUR EMOTIONAL RESPONSES HAVE YOU NOTICED OVER THIS MONTH?

Emotional patterns are like the natural rhythms of your inner landscape. Some emotions might appear predictably in certain situations, while others might cycle through in response to stress, hormonal changes, or life circumstances. Understanding these patterns helps you respond more skillfully to your emotional experience.

People who understand their emotional patterns demonstrate better mental health outcomes and more effective stress management. This awareness helps you distinguish between temporary emotional states and longer-term patterns that might need attention.

Sarah recognized subtle emotional rhythms: "Looking through my entries, I noticed that my mood consistently dipped around the third week of each month, which coincided with certain hormonal changes. Understanding this pattern helped me plan self-care during those times instead of wondering why I suddenly felt more fragile. I also noticed that my anxiety peaked on Sunday evenings, not because Sundays were bad but because I was anticipating Monday's demands."

When exploring emotional patterns, consider which emotions appeared most frequently, situations that consistently triggered similar emotional responses, times of day or days of the week when certain feelings dominated, and how long different emotions typically lasted before shifting.

Notice both challenging emotional patterns and positive ones. Perhaps you consistently feel peaceful during morning walks, energized after conversations with certain friends, or creative during quiet evening hours.

James found patterns in his emotional recovery: "I discovered that my worst depressive episodes were always followed by periods of unusual creativity and clarity. This pattern helped me understand that my emotional landscape had natural cycles rather than just being randomly difficult. When I was in the depths of sadness, I could remind myself that this state would shift, which made it more bearable."

MONTHLY DEEP DIVE PROMPT 4: HOW HAVE YOUR COPING MECHANISMS AND SELF-CARE PRACTICES DEVELOPED THIS MONTH?

Your coping strategies and self-care practices are living tools that need regular evaluation and refinement. What worked for your mental health six months ago might need adjustment based on current circumstances, new insights, or changes in your life situation.

Effective mental health management requires both reactive coping strategies for when challenges arise and proactive self-care practices that maintain your emotional baseline. This prompt helps you assess both types of tools and consider what updates might serve you better.

Sarah discovered the evolution of her self-care: "I realized my self-care had been stuck in college mode: bubble baths, face masks, and retail therapy. This month I noticed what actually restored my mental health: saying no to social plans when I needed quiet time, having real conversations instead of surface chatter, and protecting my creative energy instead of giving it away to everyone else's projects. Adult self-care looked different than I expected."

Consider which coping strategies genuinely helped during difficult moments versus those that just postponed or distracted from problems. Examine both formal techniques you've learned and informal strategies you've developed naturally.

Notice what types of self-care felt nourishing versus what felt like another obligation on your to-do list. Authentic self-care supports your well-being without creating additional stress or guilt.

James found his coping strategies maturing: "Early in my depression recovery, I thought coping meant staying constantly busy to avoid sad feelings. This month I realized that allowing myself to feel sadness without trying to fix it immediately was actually more helpful. My coping evolved from avoiding emotions to learning how to be present with them until they naturally shifted."

MONTHLY DEEP DIVE PROMPT 5: WHAT TRIGGERS OR STRESSORS CONSISTENTLY APPEARED IN YOUR LIFE THIS MONTH?

Understanding your personal triggers and stressors provides valuable information for mental health management. Some triggers might be external situations or people, while others might be internal experiences like certain thoughts, physical sensations, or emotional states.

Triggers aren't character flaws or signs of weakness. They're information about where your nervous system feels threatened or where past experiences continue to influence present reactions. Identifying patterns helps you develop appropriate responses rather than being caught off guard repeatedly.

Sarah mapped her stress triggers: "I noticed that my anxiety consistently spiked in three situations: when people asked about my plans for the future, when I had to make decisions without enough information, and when friends shared their successes right after I'd experienced setbacks. Understanding these patterns helped me prepare supportive responses instead of being overwhelmed every time these situations arose."

When exploring triggers and stressors, consider situations that repeatedly activated intense emotions, thoughts or memories that consistently disturbed your peace, physical environments or sensations that created discomfort, and relationship dynamics that regularly challenged your emotional regulation.

Notice both obvious triggers that create immediate reactions and subtler stressors that gradually build emotional charge over time. Sometimes the accumulation of small stressors creates more impact than single major events.

James identified his depression triggers: "Looking back over the month, I realized that my worst depressive episodes were often preceded by periods of social isolation, even when the isolation felt necessary at the time. Understanding this pattern helped me find ways to maintain some connection even when I needed space, which prevented isolation from spiraling into deeper depression."

MONTHLY DEEP DIVE PROMPT 6: HOW DID YOUR SOCIAL CONNECTIONS AND RELATIONSHIPS IMPACT YOUR MENTAL HEALTH THIS MONTH?

Human beings are naturally social creatures, and the quality of your relationships significantly influences your mental health. This prompt explores how different types of connection affected your emotional well-being and what patterns you might notice in your social interactions.

Social support is one of the strongest predictors of mental health resilience. However, not all social interaction provides equal benefit. Some relationships energize and support you, while others might drain your resources or trigger difficult emotions.

Sarah learned to distinguish between different types of social impact: "I assumed all social interaction was good for my mental health, but monthly reflection showed me this wasn't true. Surface-level social activities often left me feeling more isolated than before, while genuine conversations, even difficult ones, made me feel more connected to myself and others. Quality mattered more than quantity in my social life."

Consider how different relationships affected your mood, energy, and overall well-being. Notice which interactions left you feeling more yourself versus those where you felt like you needed to perform or hide parts of your experience.

Examine both the support you received from others and the support you provided. Sometimes giving meaningful help to others improves your own mental health, while other times it might deplete your resources when you're already struggling.

James found unexpected patterns in his social needs: "During my depression, I thought I needed constant social stimulation to feel better. But monthly reflection showed me that large group activities often increased my sense of isolation because I felt pressure to appear okay. One-on-one conversations with people who knew about my struggles were much more healing than trying to maintain energy for parties or big gatherings."

MONTHLY DEEP DIVE PROMPT 7: WHAT ASPECTS OF YOUR MENTAL HEALTH FELT MOST AND LEAST SUPPORTED THIS MONTH?

Mental health support comes from many sources: professional treatment, personal relationships, lifestyle choices, coping strategies, and environmental factors. This prompt helps you identify which aspects of your mental health ecosystem felt robust and which might need attention or strengthening.

Understanding what supports your mental health well helps you protect and nurture those resources. Recognizing what feels unsupported guides you toward areas where additional help or different approaches might be beneficial.

Sarah evaluated her support systems: "I realized that while I had good support for my anxiety through therapy and medication, I wasn't getting much support for my creative needs, which were closely connected to my mental health. When my creativity felt stifled, my anxiety increased. Understanding this connection helped me prioritize creative expression as part of my mental health care rather than treating it as a luxury."

Consider professional support from therapists, doctors, or other mental health providers; personal support from family, friends, or community; practical support through lifestyle, environment, or daily routines; and internal support through coping skills, self-compassion, or spiritual practices.

Notice both areas where you feel well-supported and aspects of your mental health that might benefit from additional resources or different approaches. Sometimes excellent support in one area can compensate for gaps in another.

James identified uneven support: "I had strong medical support for my depression through my psychiatrist and medication, but I realized I didn't have much emotional support for the grief that was underlying my depression. My support system was great at helping me manage symptoms but not as equipped to help me process the losses that had triggered my depression in the first place."

MONTHLY DEEP DIVE PROMPT 8: HOW DID YOUR LIFESTYLE CHOICES (SLEEP, EXERCISE, NUTRITION) AFFECT YOUR EMOTIONAL WELL-BEING THIS MONTH?

The foundation of mental health rests significantly on physical health factors. Sleep quality, movement patterns, and nutritional choices directly impact mood regulation, stress resilience, cognitive function, and emotional stability. This prompt helps you understand these connections in your own experience.

While lifestyle factors don't cure mental health conditions, they can significantly influence symptom severity and recovery speed. Understanding your personal patterns helps you make choices that support rather than undermine your emotional well-being.

Sarah tracked these connections carefully: "I discovered that my anxiety was much worse on days when I skipped breakfast or relied on coffee instead of food. I also noticed that staying up late scrolling on my phone didn't just make me tired the next day. It made me more emotionally reactive and less able to cope with normal stress. These weren't moral judgments about my choices but practical information about what my mental health needed."

Consider how different sleep patterns influenced your mood, energy, and emotional regulation. Notice what types of physical activity or movement supported your mental health versus what felt overwhelming or unsustainable.

Examine how eating patterns, meal timing, and food choices affected your emotional stability and overall well-being. Look for connections without creating rigid rules about what you should or shouldn't do.

James found that small lifestyle changes created significant mental health improvements: "I realized that my depression was significantly worse when I spent entire days indoors without natural light. Even five minutes outside in the morning made a noticeable difference in my energy and mood. Understanding this connection helped me make simple changes that supported my mental health without requiring major lifestyle overhauls."

MONTHLY DEEP DIVE PROMPT 9: WHAT LIMITING BELIEFS OR NEGATIVE SELF-TALK PATTERNS DOMINATED THIS MONTH?

Limiting beliefs and negative self-talk are like background music in your mental landscape, often unnoticed but significantly influencing your emotional experience. This prompt helps you identify repetitive thoughts that might be maintaining mental health symptoms or preventing personal growth.

Changing negative thought patterns can significantly improve mental health outcomes. However, the first step is simply becoming aware of these patterns without immediately trying to change them.

Sarah recognized her internal dialogue: "I noticed how often I used the word 'should' in my internal monologue. I should be more productive, I should handle stress better, I should be grateful instead of anxious. This constant should-ing was creating additional pressure that made my anxiety worse. I wasn't being kind to myself; I was being a harsh taskmaster disguised as self-improvement."

Common limiting beliefs include thoughts about your worthiness, capability, lovability, or safety in the world. They might sound like "I'm not good enough," "I can't handle this," "Something bad will happen," or "I'm different from everyone else."

Notice both obvious negative self-talk and subtler patterns that might seem reasonable but actually undermine your confidence or well-being. Sometimes thoughts that appear helpful or protective are actually maintaining mental health symptoms.

James identified his depression-maintaining thoughts: "I realized I was constantly telling myself stories about being a burden to others, which made me isolate and feel worse. When I started paying attention to this pattern, I could see how my depression was feeding itself through these negative stories. I wasn't ready to believe positive thoughts yet, but I could at least question whether the negative ones were actually true."

MONTHLY DEEP DIVE PROMPT 10: WHERE DID YOU EXPERIENCE THE MOST PERSONAL GROWTH IN MANAGING YOUR MENTAL HEALTH THIS MONTH?

Personal growth in mental health often appears in subtle forms that are easy to miss if you're only looking for dramatic transformations. This prompt helps you recognize real advances in emotional awareness, coping skills, relationship abilities, or overall mental health management.

Growth might look like faster recovery from difficult emotions, better recognition of your own patterns, increased willingness to seek support, improved boundary setting, or enhanced ability to distinguish between thoughts and reality. Small advances build up over time into meaningful change.

Sarah learned to appreciate gradual progress: "I expected mental health growth to feel like sudden enlightenment, but it was much more gradual. This month I noticed I was catching anxious thoughts earlier instead of letting them build into full panic. I was also asking for what I needed more directly instead of hoping people would guess. These felt like small changes, but they made daily life significantly easier."

Consider improvements in emotional regulation, relationship skills, self-compassion, or stress management. Notice increased resilience, better self-advocacy, or enhanced ability to maintain perspective during challenges.

Examine both obvious advances and subtle shifts that might be easy to overlook. Sometimes the most important growth happens in how you relate to difficulties rather than in the absence of problems.

James recognized growth in unexpected areas: "My depression symptoms weren't completely gone, but I was relating to them differently. I could feel sad without panicking about feeling sad. I could have low-energy days without deciding I was failing at life. Growth looked like developing a friendlier relationship with my own mental health rather than constantly fighting it."

MONTHLY DEEP DIVE PROMPT 11: HOW HAS YOUR UNDERSTANDING OF YOUR OWN MENTAL HEALTH NEEDS DEEPENED THIS MONTH?

Understanding your specific mental health needs, what supports your well-being, what triggers difficulties, and what helps you recover from setbacks, is an ongoing process of discovery. This prompt explores how your self-knowledge has evolved through recent experiences.

Your mental health needs might be different from what you expected or from what works for other people. Some people need more structure, others need more flexibility. Some require frequent social connection, others need substantial solitude. Learning what you specifically need helps you make choices that support rather than stress your mental health.

Sarah discovered her authentic needs: "I spent years trying to follow generic mental health advice that didn't fit my actual personality. This month I realized that meditation made my anxiety worse because sitting still amplified my worried thoughts, but walking meditation was incredibly helpful. I also learned that I need predictable routines during stressful periods and more spontaneity when life feels stable."

Consider what environments, activities, relationships, and routines genuinely support your mental health versus what you think should be helpful. Notice what timing works best for different types of self-care and when you need different types of support.

Examine how your needs might change based on circumstances, stress levels, or life transitions. What supports you during calm periods might be different from what you need during challenging times.

James learned to trust his own mental health wisdom: "I discovered that my depression recovery required a different approach than what most self-help books recommended. I needed to feel my sadness fully rather than trying to cheer myself up immediately. I needed gentle activities rather than vigorous exercise when I was struggling. Learning to trust my own experience instead of following generic advice helped me create more effective mental health strategies."

MONTHLY DEEP DIVE PROMPT 12: WHAT PROFESSIONAL OR ADDITIONAL SUPPORT FELT MOST NEEDED THIS MONTH?

Mental health is not a solo journey, and recognizing when you need additional support is a sign of wisdom rather than weakness. This prompt helps you identify what types of professional help, community resources, or other support might benefit your mental health journey.

Professional support might include therapy, psychiatry, support groups, or specialized treatment programs. Additional support could involve community resources, spiritual guidance, educational opportunities, or lifestyle changes that require expert assistance.

Sarah evaluated her support needs: "While my current therapy was helpful for anxiety management, I realized I needed additional support for the perfectionism that was underlying many of my anxious responses. I started considering whether a therapist who specialized in perfectionism might offer different tools, or whether a support group with people facing similar challenges could provide perspective my individual therapy couldn't."

Consider whether your current professional support feels adequate for your needs, what types of specialized help might address specific aspects of your mental health, whether group support or community resources could complement individual treatment, and what barriers might be preventing you from accessing helpful resources.

Notice both gaps in your current support system and areas where you feel well-supported. Sometimes adjusting existing support relationships is more helpful than adding new resources.

James recognized his changing support needs: "As my depression improved, I realized I needed different types of support. Early in recovery, I needed intensive professional help to manage symptoms. Now I needed support for rebuilding my life and relationships. This meant shifting from crisis-focused therapy to growth-oriented counseling and considering support groups for people in similar phases of recovery."

MONTHLY DEEP DIVE PROMPT 13: HOW DID MINDFULNESS, GRATITUDE, OR OTHER POSITIVE PRACTICES IMPACT YOU THIS MONTH?

Positive psychology practices like mindfulness, gratitude, appreciation, and strengths identification have substantial support for mental health improvement. This prompt explores how these practices affected your emotional well-being and which approaches felt most authentic and helpful.

Different positive practices work better for different people and at different times. Some people benefit from formal gratitude journaling, while others prefer informal appreciation of daily moments. Some find mindfulness meditation helpful, while others access present-moment awareness through movement or creative activities.

Sarah found what worked for her: "I tried gratitude lists for years because everyone said they were helpful, but they always felt forced and made me feel guilty for not being more grateful. This month I discovered that noticing small moments of beauty throughout the day, like sunlight through my kitchen window or a friend's laugh, felt more natural and actually improved my mood more than formal gratitude exercises."

Consider which positive practices felt natural and helpful versus those that felt forced or created additional pressure. Notice how different approaches to mindfulness, appreciation, or positive focus affected your mental state.

Examine both formal practices you incorporated intentionally and informal moments of presence, gratitude, or joy that arose naturally throughout your days.

James learned to adapt positive practices to his depression: "During my worst depressive episodes, gratitude practices felt toxic because they seemed to invalidate my pain. But I discovered that appreciating small comforts, like having a warm bed or a hot cup of coffee, felt authentic even when I was struggling. I had to adapt positive practices to meet me where I was rather than where I thought I should be."

MONTHLY DEEP DIVE PROMPT 14: WHAT UNRESOLVED EMOTIONS OR EXPERIENCES FROM THIS MONTH NEED ATTENTION?

Sometimes emotions or experiences require more time and space to process than daily or weekly reflection can provide. This prompt creates room for deeper exploration of situations that might still be seeking resolution or understanding.

Unresolved emotions aren't necessarily problems to solve but experiences that might benefit from additional attention, processing, or integration. They might include conflicts that ended without closure, achievements that brought unexpected feelings, losses that are still being grieved, or changes that continue to feel unsettling.

Sarah identified lingering emotional material: "I had a difficult conversation with my sister early in the month that I kept thinking about but hadn't fully processed. While the immediate conflict was resolved, I realized I was still carrying feelings about family patterns that the conversation had stirred up. These feelings weren't bad or wrong, but they needed more attention than I'd given them."

Consider situations that continue to evoke strong emotions when you remember them, achievements or changes that brought up complex feelings, relationships or interactions that feel incomplete, and decisions or transitions that still feel unsettled.

Notice both challenging emotions that might need processing and positive experiences that deserve fuller appreciation or integration. Sometimes wonderful events can bring up unexpected feelings that benefit from exploration.

James found value in processing delayed emotions: "A few weeks after starting a new medication that significantly helped my depression, I began feeling angry about how much time I'd lost to untreated symptoms. This anger was completely understandable, but I hadn't expected it and wasn't sure how to handle it. Recognizing that this delayed emotional response needed attention helped me address it appropriately instead of ignoring it."

MONTHLY DEEP DIVE PROMPT 15: HOW DO YOU WANT TO APPROACH YOUR MENTAL HEALTH DIFFERENTLY IN THE COMING MONTH?

This forward-looking prompt helps you integrate insights from monthly reflection into intentions for continued mental health growth. It's about making gentle adjustments rather than dramatic changes, building on what you've learned about yourself through recent experiences.

Effective mental health adjustments are usually small, specific, and based on actual patterns you've observed rather than generic advice or external expectations. They might involve tweaking existing practices, trying new approaches, or setting different boundaries based on what you've discovered about your needs.

Sarah set realistic intentions: "Based on this month's patterns, I realized I needed to protect my creative energy more intentionally. Instead of saying yes to every social request, I want to experiment with scheduling creative time first and then fitting social activities around it. I also want to try asking for what I need more directly instead of hoping people will guess."

Consider what insights from monthly reflection suggest practical adjustments, which patterns you'd like to shift gently, what new approaches might support your mental health, and what boundaries or intentions could guide your choices.

Focus on one or two specific changes rather than trying to overhaul everything at once. Mental health improvement happens through consistent small adjustments rather than dramatic transformations.

James planned his next steps thoughtfully: "This month showed me that I isolate when I'm stressed, which makes everything worse. Instead of trying to force myself to be social when I feel overwhelmed, I want to experiment with maintaining one small connection, maybe just texting a friend, even when I need space. I also want to continue exploring creative activities that helped my mood without pressuring myself to be productive with them."

NURTURING YOUR MONTHLY MENTAL HEALTH PRACTICE

Monthly reflection is like having a regular check-in with a wise friend who knows your whole story. Some months bring crystal-clear insights, while others offer quieter understanding that needs time to unfold. Both experiences serve your mental health journey.

Creating Sustainable Monthly Rhythm:

Choose a consistent time each month that feels spacious and supportive. This might be the first Sunday of each month, the last Friday, or any time when you can reflect without rushing or pressure.

Create a special environment for monthly reflection that feels different from your daily or weekly practice. This might involve a favorite location, comfortable seating, warm drinks, or any elements that signal this is important time for yourself.

Begin by reading through your daily and weekly entries from the past month, not to analyze everything but simply to notice what themes or patterns naturally catch your attention.

Use the monthly prompts as invitations rather than assignments. Some months, one prompt might provide rich exploration that fills your entire reflection time. Other months, you might touch on several different themes as they arise naturally.

When Monthly Reflection Feels Overwhelming:

If monthly reflection feels too emotionally intense, try focusing on just one week at a time or exploring only one prompt rather than trying to cover everything. The goal is insight and self-compassion, not comprehensive analysis.

Remember that some insights need time to develop. If a particular area feels confusing or emotionally charged, consider discussing it with a therapist, trusted friend, or support group rather than trying to process everything alone.

Moving Toward Specific Challenges

As you develop comfort with daily, weekly, and monthly mental health reflection, you might find yourself wanting tools for specific situations that arise between your regular practice times. Life doesn't always wait for scheduled reflection, and sometimes you need immediate support for particular mental health challenges.

This natural progression leads us toward situational prompts, which offer targeted guidance for those moments when anxiety strikes, depression visits, stress feels overwhelming, or any other specific mental health challenge requires immediate attention and understanding.

Your growing self-awareness through regular reflection becomes the foundation for using situational prompts effectively. You'll recognize patterns more quickly, understand your triggers more clearly, and have better tools for responding to mental health challenges as they arise.

Trust the wisdom you've developed through consistent practice as we explore these targeted tools for life's most challenging mental health moments.

FIVE
SITUATIONAL PROMPTS

Y ou know those moments in life that seem to ask something special from your mental health toolkit? Maybe it's when anxiety suddenly grips your chest during a normal day, or when depression settles over you like a heavy blanket. Perhaps it's those times when stress feels overwhelming, or when you're building resilience after a difficult experience.

Think of situational prompts as trusted companions who understand these challenging moments. They're different from your daily mental health check-ins, which help you notice regular patterns, your weekly reflections, which reveal broader themes, or even your monthly deep dives, which illuminate entire seasons of growth. These prompts are more like having a wise therapist with you when life presents specific mental health challenges that need immediate attention and understanding.

MEETING MENTAL HEALTH CHALLENGES WITH EVIDENCE-BASED WISDOM

Different mental health conditions respond better to specific therapeutic approaches. The situational prompts in this chapter draw from evidence-based treatments like Cognitive Behavioral Therapy (CBT), Dialectical Behavior Therapy (DBT), mindfulness-based approaches, and trauma-informed care. Each category includes safety protocols developed from clinical practice on therapeutic writing.

Evidence-Based Effectiveness by Condition:

Anxiety disorders show approximately 9% symptom reduction through structured writing interventions, with the strongest evidence for generalized anxiety and social anxiety. PTSD and trauma-related conditions demonstrate that about 8 out of 10 people show meaningful improvement when proper safety protocols are followed and professional supervision is available. Depression presents more complex results, with writing interventions working better as adjunct treatments rather than stand-alone approaches.

Emotional regulation challenges respond well to DBT-based journaling techniques, showing 80% compliance rates and significant improvements in emotional stability. Stress management benefits from writing interventions when integrated with mindfulness and other coping skills training.

Sarah discovered these prompts during an unexpected anxiety spiral: "I was having a panic attack in my car after a difficult meeting, feeling completely overwhelmed. Instead of fighting the feeling or trying to push through it, I remembered the prompt about anxiety in the body. Pulling out my phone to write just a few sentences about where I felt the anxiety and what it needed from me helped me ground myself. The prompt didn't make the anxiety disappear, but it gave me something concrete to do that actually helped."

James found these prompts valuable during depressive episodes: "What I love about these prompts is how they meet you exactly where you are. When depression made everything feel impossible, I didn't need inspiration or motivation. I needed gentle questions that helped me understand what was happening without judgment. These prompts became like having a compassionate therapist available whenever I needed support."

UNDERSTANDING LIFE'S MENTAL HEALTH MOMENTS

Before we explore specific situational prompts, it's important to understand when they're most helpful and when professional support might be needed instead. These prompts are designed for mental health challenges that fall within normal ranges of human experience, not for crisis situations or severe symptoms that require immediate professional intervention.

When Situational Prompts Are Helpful:

Use these prompts when you're experiencing mild to moderate symptoms that don't interfere with basic functioning, when you have mental health challenges that are familiar and manageable, when you need additional support between therapy sessions, or when you want to better understand patterns in your mental health responses.

When Professional Help Is Needed Instead:

Seek immediate professional support if you're having thoughts of self-harm or suicide, experiencing symptoms that significantly interfere with work, relationships, or daily functioning, feeling overwhelmed by emotions that don't respond to your usual coping strategies, or dealing with trauma within the past six months without professional guidance.

Each category of situational prompts includes specific safety protocols and warning signs that indicate when to stop writing and seek professional help instead.

WHEN ANXIETY STRIKES

Anxiety disorders affect millions of people and respond well to structured writing interventions when appropriate safety measures are in place. These ten prompts draw from cognitive behavioral therapy techniques and mindfulness-based approaches that have strong support.

Situational Prompt 1: When anxiety feels overwhelming in your body, where do you feel it and what does it need from you?

Anxiety often manifests as physical sensations before you consciously recognize worried thoughts. This prompt helps you develop body awareness that can provide early warning systems and grounding techniques for managing anxiety more effectively.

Focus on specific physical sensations like tightness, heat, rapid heartbeat, or shallow breathing. Notice where anxiety lives in your body and what movements, breathing patterns, or comfort measures help calm your nervous system.

Safety Protocol: If physical anxiety symptoms include chest pain, difficulty breathing, or other concerning symptoms, seek medical attention. If writing about body sensations increases panic, stop and use grounding techniques like deep breathing or progressive muscle relaxation.

Situational Prompt 2: When worrying thoughts spiral, what grounding techniques help you return to the present?

Worry spirals happen when anxious thoughts feed on themselves, creating cycles of escalating fear about future events. This prompt helps you identify and practice grounding techniques that interrupt rumination and return your attention to the present moment.

Grounding techniques can significantly reduce anxiety symptoms by activating your parasympathetic nervous system. Effective techniques might include sensory grounding (5-4-3-2-1 technique), breathing exercises, movement, or mindfulness practices.

Situational Prompt 3: When anticipatory anxiety about future events takes over, what helps you distinguish between realistic concerns and anxiety-driven fears?

Anticipatory anxiety often involves worrying about future events that may never happen or imagining worst-case scenarios that are statistically unlikely. This prompt draws from CBT techniques for examining thought accuracy and probability.

Explore what specific future events trigger your anxiety, what evidence supports or contradicts your worried predictions, what you can realistically control versus what's outside your influence, and what would constitute realistic preparation versus anxiety-driven over-preparation.

Situational Prompt 4: When social anxiety makes connection feel scary, what would self-compassion tell you?

Social anxiety often involves harsh self-criticism and predictions about negative judgment from others. This prompt applies self-compassion techniques to social fears, helping you develop a kinder internal dialogue about social interactions.

Consider what fears arise in social situations, what your inner critic tells you about others' perceptions, what you would tell a friend experiencing similar social anxiety, and what small steps toward connection feel manageable rather than overwhelming.

Situational Prompt 5: When perfectionism fuels your anxiety, what would "good enough" look like?

Perfectionism often masks anxiety about failure, rejection, or not meeting expectations. This prompt helps you explore what genuinely needs high standards versus where "good enough" would actually serve you better.

Perfectionism is strongly linked to anxiety disorders. Learning to identify when perfectionism protects you versus when it creates unnecessary stress supports better mental health outcomes.

Situational Prompt 6: When anxiety makes decisions feel impossible, what small step could you take?

Anxiety can create analysis paralysis, where the fear of making wrong choices prevents any decision-making at all. This prompt focuses on breaking decisions into manageable steps rather than requiring perfect choices.

Explore what specifically feels scary about making decisions, what information you actually need versus what anxiety tells you you need, what the smallest possible step forward would look like, and what you can learn from taking action even if it's not perfect.

Situational Prompt 7: When panic symptoms arise, what self-talk helps you remember this feeling will pass?

Panic attacks involve intense physical symptoms that can feel life-threatening even when they're not dangerous. This prompt helps you develop supportive self-talk that can provide comfort during panic episodes.

Focus on reminders that panic attacks are temporary, self-talk that normalizes rather than catastrophizes symptoms, breathing or movement techniques that help manage physical sensations, and ways to stay present during intense anxiety.

Safety Protocol: If panic symptoms include chest pain, dizziness, or other concerning physical symptoms, seek medical evaluation to rule out other conditions. If panic attacks are frequent or severe, work with a mental health professional.

Situational Prompt 8: When anxiety attacks your self-worth, what evidence contradicts these harsh thoughts?

Anxiety often generates thoughts that undermine self-confidence and self-worth. This prompt applies cognitive restructuring techniques to challenge anxiety-driven negative self-evaluation.

Examine what specific thoughts arise when anxiety affects your self-image, what evidence contradicts these negative thoughts, what friends or family might say about your worth, and what strengths you demonstrate even while managing anxiety.

Situational Prompt 9: When generalized worry consumes your day, what boundaries can you set with anxious thoughts?

Generalized anxiety disorder involves persistent worry about multiple life areas. This prompt helps you set mental boundaries with worry rather than trying to eliminate anxious thoughts entirely.

Consider what time limits you could set for worrying, what specific times of day you could designate for problem-solving versus worry, what activities help redirect your attention from anxious thoughts, and what worry thoughts deserve attention versus which ones need to be released.

Situational Prompt 10: When anxiety disrupts your sleep, what bedtime routine would support your nervous system?

Sleep disturbances are common with anxiety disorders and can create cycles where poor sleep increases anxiety, which further disrupts sleep. This prompt focuses on sleep hygiene specifically designed for anxious nervous systems.

Explore what thoughts or worries typically interfere with sleep, what physical sensations need attention before bed, what activities help calm your mind in the evening, and what environmental changes might support better sleep quality.

WHEN DEPRESSION VISITS

Depression affects millions of people worldwide and benefits from specific writing approaches that acknowledge the unique challenges of low motivation, negative thinking patterns, and emotional numbness. These prompts are designed to be gentle and accessible even during difficult periods.

Situational Prompt 11: When depression makes everything feel heavy, what tiny spark of light can you notice?

Depression often creates a lens that filters out positive experiences, making everything appear dark or meaningless. This prompt isn't about forced positivity but about gently training attention to notice small moments of comfort, beauty, or peace that exist even during difficult times.

Look for tiny comforts like warm sunlight, a pet's affection, a favorite song, or the taste of something pleasant. These sparks don't need to eliminate depression but can provide small anchors during heavy emotional weather.

Situational Prompt 12: When motivation feels absent, what is the smallest possible step toward self-care?

Depression often depletes motivation and energy, making normal self-care feel impossible. This prompt focuses on breaking self-care into the tiniest possible steps that feel manageable even during low-energy periods.

Consider what self-care needs feel most urgent, what the absolute smallest step toward meeting those needs would look like, what obstacles typically interfere with self-care, and what support might make basic care more accessible.

Situational Prompt 13: When negative self-talk dominates, what would you tell a dear friend in your situation?

Depression often amplifies self-criticism and negative self-evaluation. This prompt applies the "best friend" technique from cognitive therapy, helping you access compassion for yourself by imagining how you'd treat a friend experiencing similar struggles.

Write what specific negative thoughts are prominent, how these thoughts make you feel about yourself, what you would tell a friend who shared these same struggles, and how you might begin treating yourself with similar compassion.

Situational Prompt 14: When isolation feels safer than connection, what gentle way could you reach out?

Depression often creates urges to withdraw from relationships, which can worsen symptoms over time. This prompt explores very small steps toward connection that honor your need for space while preventing complete isolation.

Consider what feels scary about connection right now, what type of contact feels most manageable, what support you might need from others, and what boundaries would make social interaction feel safer.

Situational Prompt 15: When hopelessness clouds your vision, what has helped you through darkness before?

Depression can create cognitive distortions that make current struggles feel permanent and unsolvable. This prompt helps you access memories of resilience and recovery to provide hope during current difficulties.

Explore what previous difficult periods you've survived, what resources or strategies helped during those times, what strengths you demonstrated in past challenges, and what reminders might help you trust in your ability to get through current struggles.

Situational Prompt 16: When depression tells you nothing matters, what small things actually do bring meaning?

Depression often distorts perspective, making previously mean-ingful activities feel pointless. This prompt helps you identify small sources of meaning that persist even during depressive episodes.

Look for tiny moments of connection, simple acts of care for yourself or others, small creative expressions, or basic accom-plishments that retain some sense of purpose even when larger goals feel impossible.

Situational Prompt 17: When energy feels depleted, how can you honor your need for rest without judgment?

Depression often involves fatigue that goes beyond normal tired-ness. This prompt helps you distinguish between rest that supports healing versus isolation that maintains depression symptoms.

Consider what your body and mind actually need right now, how you can rest without guilt or shame, what activities feel restorative versus draining, and how to balance rest with gentle movement toward recovery.

Situational Prompt 18: When depression makes decisions feel overwhelming, what support do you need?

Depression can impair decision-making abilities, making choices feel overwhelming or impossible. This prompt focuses on identi-fying what support would help you navigate decisions during depressive episodes.

Explore what specifically feels difficult about making decisions, what information or perspective might help clarify choices, what support people could offer, and what decisions could be post-poned versus which ones need immediate attention.

Situational Prompt 19: When numbness replaces feeling, what gentle ways can you reconnect with sensation?

Emotional numbness is a common depression symptom where feelings become muted or absent entirely. This prompt suggests gentle approaches to reconnecting with emotional and physical sensation without forcing intense feelings.

Consider what physical sensations you can notice right now, what activities sometimes help you feel more present, what emotions feel safely accessible, and what pace of emotional reconnection feels manageable.

Situational Prompt 20: When depression whispers lies about your worth, what truths counter these messages?

Depression often generates thoughts that attack self-worth and personal value. This prompt helps you identify and strengthen truthful perspectives that counter depression's negative messaging about your worth as a person.

Write what depression tells you about your value, what evidence contradicts these negative messages, what people in your life appreciate about you, and what contributions you make that have worth regardless of your mood state.

MANAGING STRESS AND OVERWHELM

Stress management through writing can be particularly effective when combined with practical coping strategies. These eight prompts focus on both emotional processing and practical stress reduction techniques.

Situational Prompt 21: When stress feels unmanageable, what can you control versus what you need to release?

Overwhelming stress often involves trying to control things that are outside your influence while neglecting areas where you do have power. This prompt helps distinguish between effective action and energy-wasting worry.

List current stressors and categorize them into what you can directly influence, what you can partially influence, and what is completely outside your control. Focus your energy on the areas where action is actually possible.

Situational Prompt 22: When overwhelm paralyzes your thinking, what helps you break tasks into manageable pieces?

Overwhelm often happens when multiple demands feel equally urgent and impossible to prioritize. This prompt applies task management principles to reduce cognitive load and create actionable steps.

Identify what specifically feels overwhelming, how tasks could be broken into smaller components, what would need to happen for you to feel more manageable stress levels, and what support might help you organize current demands.

Situational Prompt 23: When stress manifests in your body, what movement or breathing practice brings relief?

Stress creates physical tension that can be addressed through movement and breathing techniques. This prompt helps you identify body-based stress relief that works for your specific stress patterns.

Notice where stress appears in your body, what movements help release physical tension, what breathing patterns calm your nervous system, and what environmental changes support physical stress relief.

Situational Prompt 24: When multiple stressors pile up, how can you prioritize without guilt?

Multiple stressors competing for attention can create guilt about not handling everything perfectly. This prompt provides a structure for prioritizing that reduces rather than increases stress.

List current stressors and their urgency levels, identify which stressors align with your core values, consider what consequences are acceptable versus unacceptable, and practice releasing guilt about what must be postponed or declined.

Situational Prompt 25: When stress disrupts your usual coping, what emergency self-care tools do you need?

High stress can overwhelm normal coping strategies, requiring backup approaches that work under pressure. This prompt helps you identify stress-specific self-care that remains accessible during difficult periods.

Consider what self-care typically helps you but feels impossible when stressed, what simplified versions of self-care might work during stressful periods, what emergency comfort measures you could access quickly, and what preparation might help you cope with future stress.

Situational Prompt 26: When feeling stretched too thin, what boundaries would protect your mental energy?

Chronic stress often involves taking on more than you can reasonably handle. This prompt focuses on protective boundaries that preserve mental energy for essential priorities.

Identify what demands are draining your mental energy, what boundaries would protect your capacity, what you might need to say no to, and how to communicate limits without guilt or excessive explanation.

Situational Prompt 27: When stress triggers old trauma responses, what helps you feel safe in your body?

For people with trauma histories, stress can activate old survival responses that feel disproportionate to current situations. This prompt provides gentle approaches to nervous system regulation.

Safety Protocol: If trauma responses feel overwhelming or include flashbacks, dissociation, or other severe symptoms, seek professional support. This prompt is for mild activation only.

Notice what current stress reminds your body of from past experiences, what helps you feel grounded in the present moment, what safety cues help calm your nervous system, and what professional support might help with trauma-related stress responses.

Situational Prompt 28: When chronic stress becomes your norm, what small changes could restore balance?

Long-term stress can become so familiar that it feels normal, making it difficult to recognize when stress levels are actually unhealthy. This prompt helps identify small adjustments that can begin restoring balance.

Consider how long you've been operating under current stress levels, what aspects of your life feel most out of balance, what small changes might begin shifting stress patterns, and what would help you recognize when stress levels are becoming unhealthy.

EMOTIONAL REGULATION CHALLENGES

Emotional regulation difficulties can arise from various causes and respond well to specific therapeutic approaches. These eight prompts draw primarily from Dialectical Behavior Therapy (DBT) techniques for managing intense emotions.

Situational Prompt 29: When emotions feel too big to handle, what helps you ride the wave without drowning?

Intense emotions are temporary experiences that naturally rise and fall if we don't interfere with their process. This prompt teaches "wave riding" techniques that help you tolerate intense feelings without being overwhelmed by them.

Emotions typically peak and begin subsiding within 20 to 90 seconds if we don't feed them with additional thoughts or resistance. Learning to surf emotional waves rather than fighting them improves emotional regulation.

Situational Prompt 30: When anger surprises you with its intensity, what is it trying to protect or communicate?

Anger often carries important information about boundaries, values, or unmet needs. This prompt helps you understand anger as communication rather than simply a problem to eliminate.

Explore what situation triggered your anger, what values or boundaries feel threatened, what you might need that you're not receiving, and what appropriate action your anger might be pointing toward.

Situational Prompt 31: When sadness feels endless, what reminder of impermanence brings comfort?

Intense sadness can feel permanent when you're in the middle of it. This prompt provides perspectives on emotional impermanence that can offer comfort during difficult periods without minimizing your pain.

Consider what this sadness is about, what losses or changes you might be processing, what has helped you through sadness before, and what reminders that this feeling will shift bring comfort rather than dismissal of your experience.

Situational Prompt 32: When emotions change rapidly, what anchors help you stay grounded?

Rapid emotional changes can feel disorienting and overwhelming. This prompt helps you identify stabilizing practices that provide continuity during emotional shifts.

Notice what triggers emotional changes for you, what helps you feel stable when emotions are fluctuating, what grounding techniques work regardless of your emotional state, and what support helps during periods of emotional instability.

Situational Prompt 33: When numbness replaces feeling, what gentle practices help you reconnect?

Emotional numbness can be a protective response to overwhelming situations, but extended numbness can interfere with daily functioning. This prompt offers gentle approaches to emotional reconnection.

Safety Protocol: If numbness follows trauma or includes dissociation, work with a trauma-informed therapist rather than using self-guided approaches.

Consider what might have triggered emotional shutdown, what feels safely accessible emotionally, what physical sensations you can notice, and what very gentle steps toward feeling might be manageable.

Situational Prompt 34: When shame spirals begin, what self-compassion practices interrupt the cycle?

Shame involves harsh self-judgment that can create downward spirals of negative emotions. This prompt provides self-compassion techniques specifically designed to interrupt shame cycles.

Identify what triggered feelings of shame, what critical thoughts are prominent, what you would tell a friend experiencing similar shame, and what self-compassion practices help you treat yourself with kindness.

Situational Prompt 35: When emotions feel "wrong" or "bad," how can you practice acceptance?

Many people judge their emotions as inappropriate or problematic, which often intensifies emotional distress. This prompt teaches emotional acceptance as a regulation strategy.

Explore what emotions you're judging as wrong or bad, what messages you learned about these feelings, what it might be like to experience these emotions without judgment, and how acceptance might paradoxically help emotions shift more naturally.

Situational Prompt 36: When triggered by past experiences, what helps you distinguish past from present?

Emotional triggers can make past experiences feel present and immediate. This prompt provides grounding techniques that help you stay oriented to current reality while acknowledging triggered feelings.

Notice what current situation reminds you of past experiences, what helps you feel grounded in the present moment, what support you need when past experiences feel activated, and what professional help might be beneficial for processing past experiences.

BUILDING RESILIENCE

Resilience is the ability to bounce back from challenges while maintaining your mental health and sense of self. These seven prompts help you recognize and strengthen your natural resilience.

Situational Prompt 37: When life feels particularly challenging, what inner strengths can you draw upon?

Everyone has internal resources that have helped them survive previous difficulties. This prompt helps you identify and access these strengths during current challenges.

Consider what challenges you've successfully navigated before, what personal qualities helped you through difficult times, what values or beliefs provide strength during struggles, and what evidence exists of your ability to handle adversity.

Situational Prompt 38: When setbacks occur, how can you view them as part of growth rather than failure?

Resilient people tend to interpret setbacks as learning opportunities rather than evidence of personal failure. This prompt helps reframe setbacks in ways that support continued growth and effort.

Explore what specific setback you're experiencing, what you might learn from this experience, how this setback might contribute to your long-term growth, and what would help you maintain perspective during disappointment.

Situational Prompt 39: When change feels threatening, what helps you adapt while honoring your needs?

Change often triggers anxiety because it involves uncertainty and loss of control. This prompt helps you develop adaptive strategies that honor both your need for stability and your capacity for growth.

Consider what aspects of change feel most threatening, what you need to feel safe during transitions, what has helped you adapt to previous changes, and what support would help you navigate current changes more skillfully.

Situational Prompt 40: When you doubt your ability to cope, what evidence shows your resilience?

Self-doubt during challenges is normal, but it can undermine confidence in your ability to handle difficulties. This prompt provides evidence-based reassurance about your coping capacity.

List current challenges that feel overwhelming, recall previous difficulties you've successfully managed, identify what coping strategies you're already using, and notice what evidence exists of your strength and adaptability.

Situational Prompt 41: When support feels distant, how can you become your own best ally?

Sometimes external support isn't available when you need it most. This prompt helps you develop internal supportive resources that you can access independently.

Consider what support you're missing right now, how you can provide some of this support for yourself, what self-talk would be helpful and encouraging, and what actions would demonstrate care and support for yourself.

Situational Prompt 42: When trauma responses arise, what helps you feel empowered rather than helpless?

Trauma can create feelings of powerlessness that persist even after dangerous situations have passed. This prompt focuses on rebuilding sense of agency and empowerment.

Safety Protocol: Work with trauma-informed professionals for significant trauma responses. This prompt is for mild activation only.

Notice what triggers feelings of helplessness, what helps you feel more empowered and in control, what choices you have in your current situation, and what professional support might help with trauma recovery.

Situational Prompt 43: When facing uncertainty, what practices help you tolerate not knowing?

Uncertainty is a basic part of life, but some people struggle more than others with not knowing what will happen. This prompt teaches uncertainty tolerance as a resilience skill.

Explore what specifically feels difficult about not knowing, what helps you stay present when the future is unclear, what you can control even when outcomes are uncertain, and what practices help you find peace with uncertainty.

RELATIONSHIPS AND MENTAL HEALTH

Your relationships significantly impact your mental health, and your mental health affects your relationships. These six prompts address common relationship challenges that intersect with mental wellness.

Situational Prompt 44: When relationships trigger your mental health symptoms, what boundaries serve your healing?

Some relationships, even with people you care about, can trigger anxiety, depression, or other mental health symptoms. This prompt helps you set protective boundaries without cutting off important connections.

Identify which relationships consistently affect your mental health, what specific aspects of these relationships feel triggering, what boundaries might protect your well-being, and how to maintain connection while protecting your mental health.

Situational Prompt 45: When isolation feels necessary, how can you maintain connection while protecting your energy?

Mental health challenges sometimes require periods of reduced social interaction, but complete isolation can worsen symptoms. This prompt helps you balance solitude needs with connection benefits.

Consider why isolation feels necessary right now, what type of connection feels manageable, what energy you have available for relationships, and what support you need from others during this period.

Situational Prompt 46: When others don't understand your mental health journey, how do you maintain self-advocacy?

Not everyone will understand mental health challenges, and some people may minimize or dismiss your experience. This prompt helps you advocate for your needs without requiring others' complete understanding.

Explore what understanding you need from others, how to communicate your needs clearly, what to do when people don't understand or support your mental health needs, and how to maintain confidence in your own experience despite others' reactions.

Situational Prompt 47: When relationships feel draining, what helps you distinguish between healthy give-and-take and depletion?

All relationships involve some give and take, but some relationships consistently drain your energy without reciprocal support. This prompt helps you identify when relationship dynamics are affecting your mental health.

Notice which relationships typically energize versus drain you, what makes the difference between healthy reciprocity and one-sided giving, what boundaries might restore balance, and what support you need to maintain healthy relationship patterns.

Situational Prompt 48: When mental health impacts your relationships, how can you communicate your needs clearly?

Mental health challenges can affect your availability, mood, or capacity for relationships. This prompt helps you communicate about mental health needs without shame or over-explanation.

Consider what mental health needs affect your relationships, how to explain these needs to people who matter to you, what support you need from others, and how to maintain relationships while managing mental health challenges.

Situational Prompt 49: When family dynamics trigger old patterns, what helps you respond rather than react?

Family relationships often activate old emotional patterns that may not serve your current mental health. This prompt helps you respond consciously rather than automatically in challenging family interactions.

Identify what family dynamics consistently trigger strong reactions, what old patterns you notice yourself falling into, what would help you respond more consciously, and what boundaries might protect your mental health during family interactions.

SELF-CARE AND HEALING

Self-care is essential for mental health maintenance, but many people struggle with implementing consistent self-care practices. These six prompts address common self-care challenges.

Situational Prompt 50: When self-care feels selfish, what reminder helps you prioritize your well-being?

Many people, especially those with caregiving responsibilities, struggle with guilt about taking time for self-care. This prompt helps reframe self-care as necessary rather than selfish.

Explore what messages you learned about prioritizing your own needs, how self-care actually benefits others in your life, what would help you see self-care as necessary rather than optional, and what support you need to maintain consistent self-care.

Situational Prompt 51: When healing feels too slow, how can you honor your unique timeline?

Mental health recovery often takes longer than expected and doesn't follow linear patterns. This prompt helps you work with your natural healing pace rather than forcing faster progress.

Consider what expectations you have about healing timelines, what evidence suggests healing is happening even if slowly, what would help you be patient with your own process, and what support you need during slower periods of recovery.

Situational Prompt 52: When self-care routines feel overwhelming, what is the most essential element?

Elaborate self-care routines can become burdensome rather than supportive. This prompt helps you identify the core elements of self-care that provide the most benefit with the least effort.

List your current self-care practices and identify which ones feel nourishing versus obligatory, what the most essential self-care elements are for your mental health, what simplified self-care might look like during difficult periods, and what barriers typically interfere with self-care.

Situational Prompt 53: When you skip self-care practices, what gentle return path serves you best?

Everyone occasionally skips self-care practices, but shame about inconsistency can create cycles where brief lapses become extended abandonment of helpful routines. This prompt provides compassionate approaches to returning to self-care.

Notice what typically causes you to skip self-care, what thoughts or feelings arise when you haven't maintained self-care practices, what would help you return to self-care without shame, and what adjustments might make self-care more sustainable.

Situational Prompt 54: When healing brings up difficult emotions, how can you hold space for this process?

Mental health healing often involves processing difficult emotions that may have been suppressed or avoided. This prompt helps you navigate emotional challenges that arise during recovery.

Consider what difficult emotions have emerged during your healing process, what support helps you process challenging feelings, what reminds you that difficult emotions are part of healing, and what professional support might help with emotional processing.

Situational Prompt 55: When progress feels invisible, what small victories can you acknowledge?

Mental health progress often happens in subtle ways that are easy to miss. This prompt helps you recognize gradual improvements that build into meaningful change over time.

Identify what progress you're hoping to see, what small changes you might be overlooking, what evidence exists of improvement even if subtle, and what would help you acknowledge progress without requiring dramatic transformation.

IDENTITY AND SELF-WORTH

Mental health challenges can significantly impact how you see yourself and your sense of worth. These five prompts address identity and self-worth issues that commonly arise during mental health struggles.

Situational Prompt 56: When your sense of self feels unclear, what core values remain constant?

Mental health challenges can create confusion about identity and personal direction. This prompt helps you reconnect with stable aspects of yourself that persist regardless of emotional state.

Explore what aspects of your identity feel unclear or unstable, what values have remained important to you across different life phases, what personal qualities persist regardless of your mental health state, and what activities or relationships help you feel most like yourself.

Situational Prompt 57: When mental health challenges affect your identity, how do you separate symptoms from self?

It's common to confuse mental health symptoms with personal identity, leading to shame and reduced self-worth. This prompt helps you distinguish between temporary symptoms and your essential self.

Consider what mental health symptoms feel like parts of your identity, what evidence contradicts the idea that symptoms define you, what aspects of yourself exist independently of mental health challenges, and what would help you maintain identity separate from symptoms.

Situational Prompt 58: When comparing yourself to others triggers unworthiness, what unique gifts do you bring?

Social comparison often triggers feelings of inadequacy, especially when mental health challenges make daily functioning more difficult. This prompt focuses on recognizing your unique contributions and strengths.

Notice what comparisons typically trigger feelings of unworthiness, what unique perspectives or gifts you bring to relationships and situations, what you contribute that might not be visible to others, and what would help you focus on your own path rather than comparing to others.

Situational Prompt 59: When past mistakes haunt your self-image, how can you practice self-forgiveness?

Mental health challenges can amplify shame about past mistakes, creating cycles of self-criticism that worsen symptoms. This prompt provides approaches to self-forgiveness that support healing.

Identify what past mistakes continue to affect your self-image, what you've learned from these experiences, what you would tell a friend who made similar mistakes, and what steps toward self-forgiveness feel manageable right now.

Situational Prompt 60: When others' opinions overshadow your self-worth, what internal validation do you need?

Depending heavily on external validation for self-worth creates vulnerability when others' opinions are negative or unavailable. This prompt helps develop internal sources of self-worth that provide more stable self-esteem.

Consider whose opinions affect your self-worth most strongly, what internal evidence supports your worth regardless of others' opinions, what would help you trust your own assessment of yourself, and what support you need to develop stronger internal validation.

PROFESSIONAL HELP AND TREATMENT

Integrating therapeutic writing with professional mental health treatment can boost both approaches. These five prompts address common concerns about seeking and maintaining professional support.

Situational Prompt 61: When considering therapy or treatment, what hopes and fears arise?

Seeking professional mental health treatment can bring up complex emotions. This prompt helps you explore both hopes and concerns about professional support to make informed decisions.

Explore what hopes you have about professional treatment, what fears or concerns arise when considering therapy or other treatments, what barriers might interfere with accessing professional help, and what questions you have about mental health treatment options.

Situational Prompt 62: When medication decisions feel complex, what questions need answers?

Psychiatric medication decisions often involve weighing potential benefits against possible side effects. This prompt helps you clarify questions and concerns to discuss with healthcare providers.

Consider what questions you have about medication options, what concerns arise when thinking about psychiatric medication, what information would help you make informed decisions, and what support you need when considering or adjusting medications.

Situational Prompt 63: When therapy brings up difficult material, how can you support yourself between sessions?

Therapy often involves processing challenging emotions or memories that can feel overwhelming between sessions. This prompt provides approaches to self-support during intensive therapeutic work.

Notice what difficult material has emerged in therapy, what support helps you process challenging emotions between sessions, what self-care becomes especially important during intensive therapy periods, and what emergency support you need if therapy material feels overwhelming.

Situational Prompt 64: When progress in treatment feels slow, what patience and self-compassion do you need?

Mental health treatment often takes longer than expected and includes periods of plateau or apparent lack of progress. This prompt helps maintain motivation and hope during slower periods of treatment.

Explore what expectations you have about treatment progress, what evidence of improvement you might be overlooking, what would help you be patient with your healing process, and what support you need to maintain hope during challenging periods of treatment.

Situational Prompt 65: When treatment plans need adjustment, how can you advocate for your needs?

Mental health treatment often requires adjustments based on your response and changing needs. This prompt helps you communicate effectively with treatment providers about what's working and what needs modification.

Consider what aspects of your current treatment feel helpful versus problematic, what changes you think might improve your treatment experience, how to communicate your needs clearly to treatment providers, and what questions you want to ask about adjusting your treatment plan.

WALKING WITH THESE PROMPTS THROUGH MENTAL HEALTH CHALLENGES

These situational prompts are like having a wise companion who understands that mental health challenges require specific, gentle guidance. They're not meant to replace professional treatment but to provide additional support that bridges the gap between therapy sessions, offers tools for managing symptoms as they arise, and helps you develop deeper understanding of your own mental health patterns.

Sarah discovered how these prompts transformed her relationship with mental health challenges: "Instead of feeling helpless when anxiety or depression showed up, I had specific tools that matched what I was experiencing. The prompts didn't make difficult feelings disappear, but they gave me something constructive to do that actually helped. I felt less alone with my mental health because I had these gentle guides available whenever I needed them."

James found the prompts particularly valuable during crisis moments: "What surprised me most was how having these prompts changed my relationship with difficult mental health days. Instead of just trying to survive until the feelings passed, I could use the challenging moments to understand myself better. The prompts helped me see that even my worst mental health experiences carried information that could help my healing."

Remember that these prompts work best when used with self-compassion and realistic expectations. They're tools for support and understanding, not requirements for perfect mental health management. Some days you might write pages of insight, others just a few honest sentences. Both responses serve your mental health journey.

Trust that you have everything you need to use these prompts wisely. Your willingness to explore your mental health with curiosity and compassion is the most important tool you bring to this practice. The prompts are simply guides to help you access your own wisdom about what supports your healing and growth.

As you continue forward with these tools, remember that seeking professional help when needed is a sign of strength, not weakness. These prompts complement but never replace the human connection and specialized expertise that mental health professionals provide. Use them as bridges between professional sessions, tools for daily support, and gentle companions on your ongoing journey toward mental wellness.

SIX

FINDING YOUR WAY FORWARD

You know how sometimes the most meaningful conversations leave you feeling both satisfied and curious for more? That's often how mental health journaling works. Each insight opens new doors, each understanding leads to fresh questions, and each moment of healing invites deeper exploration into your own capacity for growth and resilience.

Looking back over these prompts and tools, you might notice how they build upon each other naturally. The daily foundation prompts help you notice the quiet signals of your mental health landscape. Weekly reflection reveals patterns in those signals, showing the themes that weave through your emotional experiences. Monthly deep dives illuminate the larger seasons of your psychological growth. And those situational prompts? They stand ready as companions for those specific moments when mental health challenges need immediate, gentle attention.

YOUR MENTAL HEALTH JOURNEY CONTINUES

Think about how a garden changes when you tend it with consistent, caring attention. Each small act of nurturing contributes to its overall flourishing, creating resilience that helps it weather both gentle rains and unexpected storms. Your therapeutic journaling practice works the same way. Every entry, whether a few honest lines or several pages of deep exploration, adds to your understanding of yourself and strengthens your capacity for mental wellness.

Sarah reflects on her journey: "When I started therapeutic journaling, I thought it would give me quick answers to fix my anxiety and perfectionism. Instead, it gave me something more valuable. A way to be with myself that felt kind and curious instead of critical and demanding. I didn't eliminate anxiety, but I learned to relate to it differently. My journal became like a wise friend who helped me understand that healing isn't about becoming perfect; it's about becoming more authentically myself."

James shares his perspective: "The biggest surprise was realizing that my depression had things to teach me. Through journaling, I stopped seeing low moods as failures and started seeing them as information about what I needed. This shift didn't cure my depression, but it made the difficult times feel more manageable and meaningful. I learned that mental health isn't about feeling good all the time; it's about developing the skills to navigate whatever feelings arise."

THE GIFTS OF REGULAR THERAPEUTIC PRACTICE

Daily moments of mental health reflection become like morning light, gently illuminating what needs attention in your emotional landscape. These brief check-ins help you notice stress before it becomes overwhelming, recognize patterns before they become problematic, and appreciate small moments of peace or joy that might otherwise go unnoticed.

Weekly pauses allow you to step back and see connections you might miss day by day. Perhaps you'll notice that your anxiety consistently spikes on Sunday evenings, or that your mood improves significantly after creative activities, or that certain relationships consistently drain your mental energy while others restore it. These patterns become valuable information for designing a life that supports rather than stresses your mental health.

Monthly deep dives give you that broader perspective, helping you understand the seasonal rhythms of your emotional well-being. You might discover that your depression tends to worsen during certain times of year, that major life transitions affect your anxiety in predictable ways, or that your coping strategies need adjustment as you grow and change.

Those situational prompts stand ready like trusted friends, offering specific support when anxiety strikes, depression visits, stress feels overwhelming, or any other mental health challenge requires immediate understanding and care. They provide evidence-based guidance that can help you navigate difficult moments with greater skill and self-compassion.

CREATING YOUR OWN WAY OF HEALING

Remember those historical figures we met at the beginning of this journey? Each one found a unique way to use writing for emotional processing and mental health support. Anne Frank's diary became a lifeline to hope during unimaginable circumstances. Maya Angelou used writing to process trauma and find her voice. Virginia Woolf documented her psychological struggles while creating literary masterpieces that still offer insight into the human experience of mental illness.

Their therapeutic writing practices were as different as their lives, yet each served a vital purpose in their mental health and personal growth. Your practice will also be uniquely yours, shaped by your specific needs, preferences, and circumstances.

You might discover that early morning reflection works best for processing anxiety before the day begins, or perhaps evening reviews feel more natural for integrating the day's emotional experiences. You might find yourself drawn to certain prompts more than others, or notice that different types of reflection serve you better during different seasons of your mental health journey.

Sarah found her rhythm through experimentation: "I learned that forcing myself to journal every day actually increased my anxiety because it became another item on my perfectionist to-do list. When I shifted to writing when I felt called to it, usually three or four times a week, the practice became nurturing instead of burdensome. I also discovered that I prefer hand-writing for emotional processing but typing when I want to explore practical problem-solving."

James developed his own approach: "I found that structured prompts work better for me during depressive episodes because they give me direction when my mind feels foggy. During stable periods, I prefer more open-ended reflection. Learning to match my journaling approach to my current mental health state made the practice much more effective and sustainable."

Trust this natural evolution in your own practice. Your relation-ship with these tools will grow and change as you do. Some phases of your mental health journey might call for daily support, others for weekly reflection, and still others for monthly review with occasional situational prompts. Let your authentic needs guide your practice rather than forcing yourself into rigid patterns.

NURTURING CONTINUOUS MENTAL WELLNESS

As you continue this journey, consider how you might weave therapeutic reflection naturally into your life in ways that support rather than stress your mental health:

Gentle Daily Moments: Let brief mental health check-ins become like taking deep breaths. Natural pauses that help you stay connected to your emotional landscape without requiring extensive time or energy.

Weekly Windows: Create comfortable rhythms for looking back over your days, noticing what patterns want your attention. This might be Sunday morning coffee with your journal, Friday afternoon reflection as the week winds down, or any consistent time that feels spacious and nurturing.

Monthly Meaning-Making: Allow these deeper reflections to help you understand the larger stories unfolding in your mental health journey. Like seasonal garden reviews, monthly reflection helps you see growth, identify what needs adjustment, and plan for the coming period with greater wisdom.

Situational Support: Keep those targeted prompts close, like wise friends ready to help you understand whatever mental health challenges arise. Whether it's anxiety, depression, stress, relationship difficulties, or any other challenge, having specific tools available provides comfort even when you don't need to use them.

THE PATH AHEAD IN MENTAL HEALTH RECOVERY

Your journal becomes more valuable over time, like a garden that grows richer with each season of mindful care. It holds your stories, witnesses your growth, and offers space for continuous discovery about what supports your mental health and what interferes with your well-being.

As your therapeutic writing practice deepens, you might find yourself noticing subtle shifts in how you meet life's emotional challenges. Perhaps you'll recognize anxiety patterns more quickly and respond with greater skill. Maybe you'll develop more compassion for yourself during difficult periods, or find that you're better able to ask for help when you need it.

People who maintain regular therapeutic writing practices often experience improved emotional regulation, better stress management, enhanced self-awareness, and stronger coping skills over time. These benefits accumulate gradually, like physical fitness that builds through consistent exercise rather than dramatic workout sessions.

Sarah noticed changes she hadn't expected: "I realize now that therapeutic journaling changed not just how I handle big mental health crises, but how I navigate daily emotional experiences. I'm quicker to notice when I'm getting overwhelmed, more willing to take breaks when I need them, and much kinder to myself when things don't go perfectly. These small shifts have made my daily life significantly more peaceful."

James found that his practice supported broader life changes: "Journaling helped me understand patterns that were affecting my mental health in ways I hadn't recognized. I realized that certain work situations consistently triggered my depression, that I needed more creative expression in my life, and that some relationships were draining my emotional resources. With this understanding, I could make gradual changes that supported my mental health instead of undermining it."

A CONTINUING CONVERSATION WITH YOUR HEALING SELF

Think of your journal as an ongoing conversation with the wisest, most compassionate part of yourself. One that grows richer and deeper over time. Like those historical journal keepers we met initially, you're creating something unique and valuable. Your journal is not just a record of your mental health journey but a map of your inner landscape, a companion for your healing, and a witness to your growth.

This conversation doesn't require perfect insights or dramatic breakthroughs. Some of the most valuable journal entries are the messy ones where you're simply trying to understand what you're feeling. Others might be practical explorations of what helps your mental health and what makes it more difficult. Still others could be celebrations of small victories or gentle processing of setbacks.

The beauty of therapeutic journaling lies not in achieving perfect mental health, which doesn't exist, but in developing a friendlier, more understanding relationship with your own psychological experience. Each honest entry contributes to this relationship, helping you become more skilled at supporting yourself through whatever mental health challenges and joys life brings.

Remember that this journey isn't about reaching a destination where mental health problems never arise. It's about building your capacity to navigate whatever does arise with greater skill, self-compassion, and wisdom. Mental health, like physical health, requires ongoing attention and care. Therapeutic journaling provides tools for that care that you can access whenever you need them.

WHEN PROFESSIONAL SUPPORT ENHANCES YOUR JOURNEY

Throughout this book, we've emphasized that therapeutic journaling works best as a complement to professional mental health care rather than a replacement for it. As your self-awareness deepens through writing, you might discover areas where professional support could enhance your healing journey.

Perhaps you'll recognize patterns that would benefit from therapy, notice symptoms that could be helped by medication, or identify trauma that needs specialized treatment. Your journal insights can actually help you communicate more effectively with mental health professionals about what you're experiencing and what types of support might be most helpful.

Sarah found that journaling prepared her for therapy: "My journal entries helped me identify specific patterns and triggers that I could discuss with my therapist. Instead of just saying 'I feel anxious,' I could share concrete examples of when anxiety showed up and what seemed to help or make it worse. This made our therapy sessions much more focused and productive."

James discovered that writing between therapy sessions extended the benefits of professional treatment: "My therapist suggested I write about our sessions and any insights that came up during the week. This helped me process our work more deeply and gave me specific things to explore in future sessions. The combination of therapy and journaling was much more powerful than either approach alone."

Trust that you have everything you need to use therapeutic writing wisely while also recognizing when additional support would serve your mental health journey. The self-awareness you've developed through journaling actually makes you a better advocate for your own mental health needs.

YOUR ONGOING MENTAL HEALTH TOOLKIT

As you move forward, remember that the tools in this book are always available to you. Unlike some mental health resources that require appointments, insurance, or special circumstances, therapeutic journaling is accessible whenever you need it. Whether you're dealing with a sudden anxiety spike, processing a difficult life change, or simply wanting to check in with your-self, these prompts and practices remain ready to support you.

Your mental health toolkit now includes:

Daily foundation prompts for regular emotional awareness, weekly reflection techniques for pattern recognition, monthly deep dive practices for broader understanding, situational prompts for specific challenges, evidence-based safety protocols to protect your well-being, and integration strategies for working with professional support.

But perhaps most importantly, you've developed the capacity to meet yourself with curiosity and compassion through writing. This skill, the ability to explore your inner experience with kind-ness rather than judgment, serves as the foundation for all other mental health tools and strategies.

KEEP WRITING, KEEP GROWING

Your journey with therapeutic journaling continues one reflec-tion at a time. Some days might bring deep insights that shift your perspective significantly. Others might offer quiet observa-tions that contribute to gradual understanding. Still others might simply provide a peaceful moment of connection with yourself. All of these experiences serve your mental health and personal growth.

Keep writing, keep wondering, and keep showing up for this gentle conversation with yourself. Each blank page offers a fresh invitation to understand your mental health more deeply, develop greater skill in supporting your own well-being, and discover what wisdom awaits in your own experience.

Trust both the evidence that supports therapeutic writing and your own intuition about what serves your mental health best.

The science provides a foundation of understanding, but your personal experience remains the ultimate guide for how these tools can best support your unique journey toward mental wellness.

Remember what we learned from those thousands of people in studies: therapeutic writing creates real, measurable improvements in mental health when used consistently and with appropriate safety measures. You're not just hoping these tools will help. You're using evidence-based practices that have supported healing for countless people dealing with anxiety, depression, stress, trauma, and other mental health challenges.

As Sarah reminds us: "Therapeutic journaling didn't solve all my mental health problems, but it gave me a way to work with them that felt empowering instead of overwhelming. I learned that I don't have to wait for someone else to understand my mental health. I can develop that understanding myself and use it to create a life that supports my well-being."

James adds: "The most important thing I learned is that mental health isn't something you achieve and then maintain forever. It's something you tend, like a garden. Some seasons require more intensive care, others allow for simply enjoying what's growing. Therapeutic journaling gave me tools for every season of my mental health journey."

Your journey continues and these tools go with you, ready to help you discover deeper understanding, greater resilience, and more effective ways of supporting your own mental wellness. Trust that you have everything you need to use them wisely, seek additional support when helpful, and continue growing in your capacity for mental health and emotional well-being.

The conversation with yourself through therapeutic writing is just beginning. Each entry you make adds to your understanding, each insight you gain strengthens your resilience, and each moment of self-compassion you practice contributes to your healing. Keep going, one reflection at a time, trusting in your own capacity for growth and the evidence-based power of therapeutic writing to support your mental health journey.

APPENDIX I. RESOURCES FOR DEEPER HEALING AND SUPPORT

You know how one meaningful conversation about mental health often leads to another, opening doors to new understanding and possibilities for healing? As your therapeutic journaling practice grows, you might find yourself curious about different approaches or wanting to explore specific aspects of mental wellness more deeply. Here are carefully chosen resources to support your ongoing journey toward emotional well-being.

BOOKS THAT SUPPORT MENTAL HEALTH THROUGH WRITING

Think of these books as wise companions for different aspects of your healing journey. Each offers unique insights into using writing as a tool for mental health support, backed by solid evidence and clinical experience.

Understanding the Power of Therapeutic Writing

"Writing to Heal" by James Pennebaker and Joshua Smyth is like having a conversation with the people who've spent decades understanding how writing transforms mental health. They share fascinating insights about why putting emotional experiences into words can be so powerful for psychological healing, along with specific approaches that have helped thousands of people process trauma, anxiety, and depression.

"The Writing Cure" by Susan Zimmermann explores how different types of writing can address various mental health challenges. Zimmermann, both a therapist and writing instructor, bridges the gap between clinical practice and creative expression, showing how structured writing exercises can complement traditional therapy.

Deepening Your Mental Health Practice

"Journal to the Self" by Kathleen Adams offers an extensive toolkit of journaling techniques specifically designed for emotional healing and personal growth. Adams, a pioneer in journal therapy, provides structured approaches for working with trauma, relationships, life transitions, and other mental health challenges through writing.

"Therapeutic Journaling" by Kay Adams (no relation to Kathleen) presents evidence-based approaches to using writing in mental health treatment. This book is particularly valuable for understanding how journaling can support recovery from depression, anxiety, PTSD, and other conditions.

"Expressive Writing: Counseling and Healthcare" by Gillie Bolton explores how healthcare providers and counselors integrate therapeutic writing into treatment. While written for professionals, it offers valuable insights for anyone wanting to understand the clinical applications of writing for mental health.

Additional Books in the Mental Health Journaling Series

"The Art of Therapeutic Journaling" provides comprehensive guidance for building strong foundations in mental health writing practice. This companion guide helps you select appropriate techniques for different symptoms, work through common barriers to therapeutic writing, and integrate journaling with mindfulness and other wellness practices.

"Anxiety Relief Through Writing" focuses specifically on using structured writing to manage anxiety disorders, panic attacks, and worry patterns. Based on cognitive behavioral therapy principles, it offers targeted exercises for challenging anxious thoughts and building emotional regulation skills.

"Depression Recovery Journaling Guide" addresses the unique challenges of maintaining a writing practice during depressive episodes, with gentle approaches that honor low-energy periods while supporting gradual healing and recovery.

"The Trauma-Informed Writing Workbook" provides specialized guidance for using writing to process traumatic experiences safely, with extensive safety protocols and integration with professional trauma treatment.

DIGITAL TOOLS FOR MENTAL HEALTH PRACTICE

While handwriting offers unique neurological benefits for therapeutic processing, digital tools can provide valuable support for mental health journaling, especially when designed with evidence-based principles and appropriate safety measures.

Evidence-Based Mental Health Journal Apps

Daylio combines mood tracking with brief journaling, allowing you to notice patterns in your emotional states over time. Mood tracking can improve emotional awareness and help identify triggers for mental health symptoms.

Journey offers a secure, private platform for therapeutic writing with features like guided prompts, mood correlation, and export capabilities that support sharing insights with mental health professionals.

Sanvello (formerly Pacifica) integrates journaling with anxiety and depression tracking, providing tools based on cognitive behavioral therapy principles along with professional content review.

Mood Tracking Integration and Outcome Monitoring

Digital platforms can boost therapeutic writing by providing visual representations of mood patterns, symptom tracking, and progress monitoring. However, make sure any app you choose includes robust privacy protections and crisis detection capabilities.

Important considerations for digital mental health tools:

Look for apps developed with mental health professionals, verify that crisis detection and support systems are available 24/7, make sure there are strong privacy protections and data security, and choose platforms that integrate with professional treatment when appropriate.

AI-Assisted Journaling: Emerging Possibilities and Applications

Recent 2024 studies show remarkable promise for AI-assisted therapeutic writing, with about 8 out of 10 people showing improvement in depression and anxiety, comparable to traditional therapy outcomes. However, AI tools require careful evaluation for safety and therapeutic appropriateness.

Criteria for evaluating AI writing tools:

Professional oversight in development and content review, clear limitations and crisis escalation protocols, integration capabilities with human mental health providers, transparent algorithms and evidence-based approaches, and strong privacy protections and ethical data use.

Privacy and Security Considerations for Digital Mental Health Tools

Mental health information is particularly sensitive and deserves the highest level of protection. When choosing digital tools for therapeutic writing, prioritize platforms that offer end-to-end encryption, clear data ownership policies, transparent privacy practices, and regulatory compliance with healthcare privacy laws.

FINDING MENTAL HEALTH COMMUNITY

Sometimes, sharing aspects of your mental health journey with others can deepen your healing while maintaining the privacy of your personal reflections. Community support provides perspective, reduces isolation, and offers encouragement during challenging periods.

Online Mental Health Journaling Groups

Reddit's r/Journaling includes many people using writing for mental health support, with subgroups focused on specific conditions like anxiety, depression, and trauma recovery. While maintaining appropriate boundaries, these communities can provide inspiration and practical tips.

International Association for Journal Writing offers online groups and workshops specifically focused on therapeutic journaling, led by trained facilitators who understand mental health applications.

7 Cups provides free emotional support through trained listeners and includes journaling features integrated with peer support networks.

Local Therapy and Support Groups

Consider looking for National Alliance on Mental Illness (NAMI) support groups that welcome journaling as part of recovery, Depression and Bipolar Support Alliance (DBSA) groups that integrate writing practices, community mental health centers offering writing therapy groups, and libraries or community centers hosting therapeutic writing workshops.

Mental Health-Focused Writing Circles

Many communities offer writing groups specifically designed for people working on mental health recovery. These groups typically focus on the therapeutic benefits of writing rather than literary critique, providing safe spaces to explore emotional topics through structured writing exercises.

What to look for in therapeutic writing groups:

Facilitators with mental health training or supervision, clear guidelines about confidentiality and safety, focus on personal healing rather than writing quality, integration with professional mental health resources, and appropriate crisis intervention protocols.

COMPLEMENTARY MENTAL HEALTH PRACTICES

Like different plants supporting each other in a garden, various practices can boost your therapeutic journaling journey and overall mental wellness.

Movement and Mental Health Therapy

Walking meditation for anxiety relief: Combining gentle movement with mindful awareness can calm an activated nervous system while providing space for insights to emerge. Many people find that solutions to problems arise naturally during mindful walking.

Yoga and therapeutic writing combinations: The body awareness developed through yoga practice can boost your ability to notice physical signals of mental health changes. Some people find that writing after yoga practice accesses deeper emotional insights.

Exercise journaling for depression management: Regular physical activity can be as effective as medication for some types of depression. Combining exercise with reflection about mood, energy, and motivation can help you understand what types of movement best support your mental health.

Handwriting Benefits: Neurological Evidence

Recent neurological studies strongly favor handwriting over typing for therapeutic benefit. Brain imaging shows that handwriting activates broader neural networks than typing, engaging visual, motor, and cognitive regions simultaneously. This enhanced brain connectivity appears to be one mechanism through which writing creates therapeutic change.

Practical implications:

Choose handwriting for emotional processing when possible, use typing for longer reflections or when handwriting isn't accessible, consider digital stylus writing as a middle ground, and trust your personal preference while understanding what the science shows.

Creative Expression for Healing

Art therapy techniques with journaling: Combining visual elements with written reflection can access emotional experiences that words alone might not reach. This might include drawing emotional states, creating collages about recovery goals, or using colors to represent different aspects of mental health.

Music and mental health reflection: Many people find that music helps them access and process emotions. Consider writing about songs that resonate with your experience, using music as a prompt for reflection, or creating playlists that support different aspects of your mental health journey.

Poetry for emotional processing: Poetic language can capture emotional experiences that prose cannot express. You don't need to be a poet to benefit from exploring feelings through imagery, metaphor, and rhythm.

MINDFULNESS PRACTICES THAT BOOST THERAPEUTIC WRITING

Mindfulness, the practice of paying attention to the present moment without judgment, significantly boosts the benefits of therapeutic writing by increasing emotional awareness and reducing reactivity.

Meditation and Therapeutic Writing

Brief meditation before writing can help you access deeper emotional awareness and reduce mental chatter that might interfere with honest reflection. Even five minutes of focusing on your breath can create helpful space for therapeutic exploration.

Mindful writing practice involves paying attention to the physical sensation of writing, noticing thoughts and feelings as they arise without immediately judging them, and staying present with whatever emotional material emerges during writing.

Body Awareness for Trauma Recovery

For people with trauma histories, developing body awareness through mindfulness can support therapeutic writing by helping you recognize when you're approaching emotional limits and need to slow down or seek additional support.

Gentle body scanning before writing can help you notice current emotional and physical states, providing important information about what kind of reflection would be most helpful in the moment.

Present Moment Practice for Anxiety

Anxiety often involves worry about future events that may never happen. Mindfulness practices that anchor attention in the present moment can provide relief from anxious rumination and create space for more balanced perspective.

Grounding techniques that engage your senses (5-4-3-2-1 technique) can be particularly helpful before therapeutic writing sessions when anxiety is present.

WHEN YOU NEED PROFESSIONAL SUPPORT

Deep therapeutic writing sometimes stirs up challenging emotions or reveals mental health needs that require professional expertise. Knowing when and how to seek additional support is an important skill that protects your well-being and boosts your healing journey.

Finding Therapists Who Support Journaling

Many mental health professionals welcome therapeutic writing as a complement to traditional therapy. When seeking professional support, consider asking potential therapists about their experience with writing interventions, their approach to homework and between-session activities, and their comfort with clients who use journaling as part of their healing process.

Types of therapy that commonly integrate writing:

Cognitive Behavioral Therapy (CBT) often includes thought records and behavioral monitoring, Dialectical Behavior Therapy (DBT) uses diary cards and mindfulness writing, narrative therapy specifically focuses on rewriting life stories, and expressive arts therapy combines writing with other creative modalities.

Crisis Resources and Hotlines

Keep these resources easily accessible in your writing space and on your phone:

National Crisis Lines:

National Suicide Prevention Lifeline: 988, Crisis Text Line: Text HOME to 741741, National Alliance on Mental Illness (NAMI): 1-800-950-NAMI

Specialized Resources:

National Sexual Assault Hotline: 1-800-656-HOPE, National Domestic Violence Hotline: 1-800-799-7233, LGBTQ National Hotline: 1-888-843-4564, Veterans Crisis Line: 1-800-273-8255

Integrating Journaling with Professional Treatment

Therapeutic writing can significantly boost professional mental health treatment when integrated thoughtfully. Many people find that journaling between therapy sessions helps them process insights more deeply and arrive at sessions with specific topics to explore.

Ways to integrate journaling with therapy:

Share relevant insights from your writing practice with your therapist, use prompts to prepare for therapy sessions by clarifying what you want to discuss, write about therapy sessions afterward to integrate new perspectives, track medication effects, side effects, and mood changes through writing, and use journaling to practice therapeutic techniques between sessions.

Collaboration protocols with treatment providers:

Discuss your writing practice with your treatment team, ask about specific writing exercises that might support your treatment goals, share pattern recognition from your journaling that might inform treatment planning, use writing to track progress toward therapy goals, and maintain appropriate boundaries about what writing content to share.

Remember that not all journal content needs to be shared with therapists. Your writing practice can maintain areas of privacy while still supporting your professional treatment through enhanced self-awareness and emotional processing.

CREATING YOUR RESOURCE GARDEN

Think of these resources as different plants in your garden of mental health recovery. Some might call for your attention right away, while others might be perfect for future seasons of growth. Trust your intuition about what supports you best right now while knowing that additional resources remain available as your needs evolve.

Sarah reflects on her resource exploration: "I started by trying everything at once, thinking more resources would create faster healing. That approach felt overwhelming and scattered. When I learned to choose one or two resources that matched my current needs and capacity, my mental health practice became much more sustainable and effective."

James found his path through gradual exploration: "I began with just therapeutic journaling and slowly added other resources as I felt ready. First, I joined an online support group. Later, I started working with a therapist who understood writing interventions. Eventually, I added mindfulness meditation and creative expression. Building my resource toolkit gradually helped me integrate each element before adding something new."

Remember that, like any good conversation about mental health, your relationship with these resources will evolve naturally. Let them inspire and support you without feeling pressure to use them all immediately. Your healing journey is unique, and you'll recognize which tools and practices feel right for different moments along the way.

The most important resource you bring to this journey is your own willingness to explore your mental health with curiosity and compassion. Everything else can be learned and adapted as you grow in understanding of what supports your unique path toward emotional well-being.

APPENDIX II. COMPREHENSIVE FOUNDATION

Isn't it fascinating how something as simple as putting pen to paper can create measurable changes in your mental health? While people have known intuitively for centuries that writing helps process emotions and find healing, modern science has revealed the specific mechanisms that make therapeutic writing so powerful for psychological wellness.

PENNEBAKER'S FOUNDATIONAL WORK: THE BIRTH OF EXPRESSIVE WRITING

In 1986, psychology professor James Pennebaker asked a simple question: What happens when people write about their deepest thoughts and feelings regarding traumatic experiences? His groundbreaking study at Southern Methodist University would change how we understand the relationship between writing and mental health.

Pennebaker divided college students into two groups. One group wrote about traumatic experiences for fifteen minutes a day over four consecutive days. The control group wrote about trivial topics like describing their shoes. What happened next surprised everyone, including Pennebaker himself.

The Original 1986 Study Results: Students who wrote about traumatic experiences visited the health center 50% less over the following six months compared to the control group. Their immune system function improved, as measured by t-lymphocyte response. Blood pressure and heart rate decreased during writing sessions. Most surprisingly, academic performance improved despite writing about difficult emotional material.

This wasn't just a temporary feel-good effect. The benefits persisted for months after the brief writing intervention ended. Pennebaker had discovered something remarkable: structured emotional expression through writing creates lasting improvements in both physical and mental health.

Development of the Optimal Protocol: Through decades of follow-up work, Pennebaker's team refined the expressive writing protocol that remains the gold standard today:

Write continuously for 15 to 20 minutes, focus on deepest thoughts and feelings about the experience, don't worry about grammar, spelling, or eloquence, write for yourself, not for others to read, and repeat for 3 to 4 sessions over consecutive days or weeks.

The Inhibition Theory: Pennebaker proposed that suppressing emotions creates physiological stress that manifests as health problems. Writing provides a safe outlet for emotional expression while helping people make meaning of difficult experiences. The combination of emotional expression and cognitive processing appears crucial for therapeutic benefit.

Linguistic Pattern Analysis: Perhaps most interesting, Pennebaker's team discovered that certain writing patterns predict better outcomes. People who show progression from disorganized to coherent narratives benefit more than those whose writing remains scattered. Increased use of causal words (because, reason) and insight words (understand, realize) correlates with better physical and mental health improvements.

META-ANALYTIC EVIDENCE: DECADES OF CONFIRMATION

Since Pennebaker's original study, hundreds of studies involving tens of thousands of participants have been conducted. Multiple meta-analyses provide robust evidence for therapeutic writing's mental health benefits.

Smyth's 1998 Meta-Analysis: Dr. Joshua Smyth analyzed 13 major studies involving 2,085 participants. About 7 out of 10 people who engaged in expressive writing showed better outcomes than control groups across multiple measures of mental and physical health.

Frattaroli's 2006 Comprehensive Review: Dr. Stefanie Frattaroli examined 146 studies with 20,423 participants, providing the most comprehensive analysis to date. While the overall effect was smaller, it remained statistically significant across this massive dataset. The consistency of findings across diverse populations and conditions tells a compelling story about writing's therapeutic potential.

Recent Analyses (2020-2024): Contemporary meta-analyses continue to show consistent small to moderate effects for expressive writing interventions. However, scientists have identified important factors that explain why some people benefit more than others:

Number of sessions: Three or more sessions show significantly better outcomes than single sessions. Writing environment: Private, secure settings boost therapeutic benefits. Specific instructions: Structured prompts outperform completely free writing. Individual differences: Emotional expressiveness and baseline stress levels influence outcomes. Cultural factors: Most studies involve Western populations; adaptation may be needed for other cultures.

NEUROBIOLOGICAL MECHANISMS: HOW WRITING CHANGES YOUR BRAIN

Recent advances in neuroimaging technology have revealed exactly how therapeutic writing affects brain function. These discoveries help explain why writing can be so powerful for mental health recovery and maintenance.

Brain Connectivity: 2024 studies using functional magnetic resonance imaging (fMRI) show that handwriting activates broader neural networks than typing. When you write by hand, visual, motor, and cognitive brain regions work together in ways that don't occur during typing. This enhanced connectivity may explain why handwriting often feels more therapeutic than digital journaling.

Specific brain regions affected by therapeutic writing include:

Prefrontal cortex: Enhanced activation improves emotional regulation and impulse control. Anterior cingulate cortex: Better integration of emotional and cognitive processing. Hippocampus: Improved memory consolidation and trauma processing. Amygdala: Reduced reactivity to emotional triggers over time.

Stress Response Regulation: Therapeutic writing creates measurable changes in your body's stress response system:

Cortisol reduction: Lower levels of the primary stress hormone. HPA axis regulation: Better communication between brain and adrenal glands. Autonomic balance: Improved heart rate variability indicating better stress resilience. Inflammation markers: Decreased levels of inflammatory proteins linked to depression and anxiety.

Working Memory and Emotional Processing: Writing appears to free up cognitive resources by transferring emotional material from working memory to paper. This explains why people often report feeling "lighter" after therapeutic writing sessions. Your brain literally has more capacity for problem-solving and emotional regulation when difficult experiences are externalized through writing.

EVIDENCE BY MENTAL HEALTH CONDITION

Different mental health challenges respond differently to writing interventions. Understanding the specific findings for each condition helps set realistic expectations and choose appropriate approaches.

Anxiety Disorders: Consistent Moderate Benefits

Generalized Anxiety Disorder (GAD): A meta-analysis of 20 randomized controlled trials found that structured writing interventions produce an average 9% reduction in anxiety symptoms. While this might sound modest, it represents meaningful relief for daily functioning and quality of life.

Social Anxiety: Limited direct studies exist for social anxiety and writing interventions. However, CBT-based writing exercises that challenge social fears and catastrophic thinking show promise when combined with gradual exposure to social situations.

Panic Disorder: Writing interventions that focus on understanding panic triggers, tracking symptoms, and challenging catastrophic interpretations of physical sensations can reduce panic frequency and intensity. However, this works best as an adjunct to professional treatment rather than a standalone intervention.

PTSD and Trauma: Strong Evidence with Important Caveats

Written Exposure Therapy: Studies show that structured writing about traumatic experiences can be as effective as traditional trauma therapies when conducted with proper safety protocols. About 8 out of 10 people show meaningful improvement.

Critical Safety Considerations:

Not recommended within 6 months of acute trauma, requires professional supervision for complex trauma, contraindicated for people with high dissociation, and should not be attempted during active crisis periods.

Cognitive Processing Therapy (CPT): Studies show that cognitive-only approaches to trauma recovery can be as effective as written trauma accounts for most patients. This suggests that challenging trauma-related beliefs through writing may be the active ingredient rather than simply recounting traumatic events.

Depression: Mixed Results Requiring Nuanced Understanding

Major Depressive Disorder: Studies on expressive writing alone for depression show mixed results. Some studies find no significant long-term effects, while others show modest improvements. The key appears to be combining writing with other therapeutic approaches rather than using it as a standalone treatment.

Gratitude Journaling: Specific forms of positive writing show more consistent benefits for depression. Gratitude journaling helps about 1 in 5 people feel noticeably better about their lives. However, gratitude practices may feel inauthentic or counterproductive during severe depressive episodes.

Behavioral Activation Through Writing: Writing interventions that focus on planning and reflecting on meaningful activities show better outcomes for depression than purely expressive writing. This suggests that structured problem-solving through writing may be more helpful than emotional expression alone for depressive symptoms.

Emotional Regulation: Strong Evidence from DBT Practice

Dialectical Behavior Therapy (DBT) Diary Cards: Studies on DBT diary techniques show remarkable results for emotional regulation problems:

80% average compliance rate with daily emotion tracking, significant improvements in affective instability and identity problems, reduced self-harm behaviors when combined with professional DBT treatment, and better medication compliance and therapy engagement.

Emotion Labeling Through Writing: Studies show that simply naming emotions accurately through writing can reduce their intensity. This "affect labeling" activates prefrontal brain regions that help regulate emotional responses. The more specific your emotional vocabulary, the better your emotional regulation becomes.

THERAPEUTIC INTEGRATION EVIDENCE

Understanding how writing interventions integrate with established therapeutic approaches helps maximize their effectiveness while maintaining safety.

Cognitive Behavioral Therapy (CBT) Integration

Thought Records: Studies consistently show high effectiveness for written thought challenging exercises. CBT-based writing helps people:

Identify cognitive distortions more systematically, develop balanced thinking patterns, practice cognitive restructuring between therapy sessions, and track progress in challenging negative thought patterns.

Behavioral Experiments: Writing about planned behavioral experiments and their outcomes boosts the learning process. Studies show that written reflection on exposure exercises and behavioral changes increases their therapeutic impact.

Homework Compliance: Studies indicate significantly higher homework completion rates when CBT assignments involve writing components. The act of writing seems to increase engagement and retention of therapeutic techniques.

Acceptance and Commitment Therapy (ACT) Based Writing

Values Clarification: Studies show that writing exercises focused on identifying and connecting with personal values create superior outcomes for psychological flexibility, a key component of mental health according to ACT theory.

Mindful Writing Practices: Studies on mindful journaling show benefits for:

Present-moment awareness, acceptance of difficult emotions, reduced experiential avoidance, and better commitment to value-based actions.

Defusion Techniques: Writing exercises that help people relate differently to thoughts (seeing thoughts as mental events rather than absolute truths) show promising results for anxiety, depression, and stress management.

Trauma-Informed Approaches

Window of Tolerance Considerations: Studies emphasize the importance of maintaining emotional regulation during trauma-focused writing. People need to stay within their "window of tolerance," neither numb nor overwhelmed, for writing to be therapeutic rather than retraumatizing.

Clinic-Based vs. Self-Guided: Studies show that trauma-focused writing works best when conducted in clinical settings with professional supervision. Self-guided trauma writing can be beneficial for minor stressors but should be avoided for significant trauma without professional support.

Phase-Oriented Treatment: Studies support a gradual approach to trauma writing that begins with safety and stabilization before moving to trauma processing. This aligns with established trauma treatment protocols that prioritize safety above emotional expression.

OPTIMAL PRACTICE PARAMETERS: WHAT WE KNOW

Decades of studies have identified specific parameters that maximize therapeutic writing's mental health benefits while minimizing potential risks.

Frequency and Duration: The Goldilocks Principle

Minimum Effective Dose: Studies consistently show that 3 sessions of 15 minutes each represents the minimum effective dose for therapeutic writing benefits. Shorter interventions may provide temporary relief but don't create lasting change.

Optimal Protocol: The most studied and effective protocol involves:

15 to 20 minutes per session, 3 to 4 sessions total, sessions spaced over consecutive days or 3 times weekly, focus on thoughts AND feelings, not just events, and private, secure writing environment.

Intervention Length: Studies show that benefits continue to accrue with practice over 30+ days. However, most studies focus on short-term interventions (1-4 weeks). Long-term studies suggest that periodic "booster" writing sessions help maintain benefits.

Diminishing Returns: Interestingly, studies suggest that more isn't always better. Sessions longer than 30 minutes may become overwhelming, while daily writing for extended periods can sometimes increase rumination rather than provide relief.

Safety and Contraindications: Critical Findings

Contraindicated Populations: Studies identify several groups for whom unsupervised expressive writing may be problematic:

Alexithymia: People with difficulty identifying emotions may find expressive writing frustrating and unhelpful. Active psychosis: Reality testing problems make unsupervised writing potentially dangerous. Recent acute trauma: Writing about trauma within 6 months requires professional supervision. High dissociation: People prone to dissociative responses need specialized trauma-informed approaches.

Warning Signs from Studies: Studies help identify concerning responses that require professional intervention:

Immediate distress lasting more than 2 hours after writing, increased rumination without cognitive processing or insight, compulsive writing behaviors that feel out of control, and deteriorating mental health that coincides with writing practice.

Protective Factors: Studies identify elements that boost safety:

Time limits (20-minute maximum sessions), structured prompts rather than completely free writing, regular emotional check-ins during and after writing, easy access to professional support when needed, and clear understanding of when to stop and seek help.

Special Populations: Considerations

Age Factors:

Adolescents: Show small but significant benefits with appropriate supervision. Older adults: Mixed findings; reminiscence-based approaches may work better than problem-focused writing. Children: Limited studies; requires specialized approaches and professional guidance.

Cultural Considerations:

Most studies conducted with white, educated, Western populations. Collectivist cultures may require adapted approaches that honor family and community perspectives. Language and emotional expression norms vary significantly across cultures. Individual vs. community healing approaches may need adjustment.

Clinical Populations:

Severe mental illness: Requires professional supervision and integration with comprehensive treatment. Substance use disorders: Shows promise when combined with addiction treatment programs. Eating disorders: Mixed results; may need specialized approaches to avoid triggering restrictive behaviors.

COMPARATIVE EFFECTIVENESS: HOW WRITING STACKS UP

Understanding how therapeutic writing compares to other mental health interventions helps set realistic expectations and inform treatment decisions.

Writing vs. Traditional Psychotherapy

Enhanced Expressive Writing: Studies show that when expressive writing includes brief therapist contact, outcomes approach those of traditional psychotherapy for trauma recovery. This suggests that minimal professional support can significantly boost writing's therapeutic potential.

Standalone vs. Therapist-Guided: Studies indicate that self-guided expressive writing achieves approximately 75-80% of the effectiveness of therapist-guided approaches for appropriate populations. This makes writing an incredibly cost-effective intervention for many mental health challenges.

Cost-Effectiveness Analysis: Economic studies show remarkable cost-effectiveness for writing interventions:

Cost per participant: $0-50 (compared to $100-200 per therapy session), significant healthcare cost reductions through improved physical health, reduced need for crisis interventions when used appropriately, and scalable to large populations through digital platforms.

Writing vs. Medication

Complementary Rather Than Competitive: Studies don't position writing as an alternative to psychiatric medication but as a valuable complement. Studies show that people who combine medication with therapeutic writing often achieve better outcomes than either intervention alone.

Specific Comparisons:

Antidepressants: Writing doesn't replace medication for moderate to severe depression but may boost treatment response and reduce relapse rates. Anti-anxiety medications: Writing may help reduce reliance on PRN (as-needed) anxiety medications by providing alternative coping tools. Sleep medications: Some studies suggest that evening reflective writing can improve sleep quality, potentially reducing need for sleep aids.

Format Comparisons: What Works Best

Handwriting vs. Typing: Neurological studies strongly favor handwriting for therapeutic benefit:

Broader neural network activation, enhanced memory consolidation, greater emotional engagement, and better integration of cognitive and emotional processing.

Structured vs. Unstructured Writing: Studies consistently show that structured prompts outperform completely free writing:

Provide direction when emotions feel overwhelming, help access specific therapeutic techniques, reduce rumination and increase insight, and offer safety through contained exploration.

Positive vs. Expressive Writing: Different approaches work better for different populations:

Expressive writing: More effective for trauma, anxiety, and stress. Positive writing: Better for general mood improvement and life satisfaction. Combined approaches: May offer benefits of both without overwhelming vulnerable populations.

EMERGING POSSIBILITIES AND FUTURE DIRECTIONS

The field of therapeutic writing continues to evolve, with exciting developments in technology, personalization, and our understanding of biological mechanisms.

AI-Assisted Journaling: Breakthrough 2024 Studies

First Randomized Controlled Trial: A groundbreaking 2024 study of AI-assisted therapeutic journaling produced remarkable results:

Depression improvements: About 8 out of 10 people showed meaningful improvement. Anxiety reduction: Similar rates of improvement. Therapeutic alliance: User ratings comparable to human therapists. Safety outcomes: No adverse events with proper crisis detection protocols.

How AI Enhancement Works:

Personalized prompts based on previous entries, real-time emotional support and validation, crisis detection and immediate human intervention when needed, progress tracking and pattern recognition, and integration with human therapists when appropriate.

Future Implications: This study suggests that well-designed AI systems could dramatically expand access to therapeutic writing support while maintaining safety and effectiveness. However, ethical considerations about data privacy, algorithm transparency, and appropriate limitations remain crucial.

Digital Platform Safety Standards

Crisis Detection Requirements: Studies identify essential safety features for digital therapeutic writing platforms:

24/7 crisis detection and response capabilities, immediate escalation to human professionals when needed, clear limitations about what AI can and cannot provide, integration with local emergency services, and comprehensive privacy and data protection.

Quality Standards: Emerging studies suggest standards for evaluating digital mental health writing tools:

Professional oversight in development and content review, evidence-based approaches with published support, transparent algorithms and decision-making processes, regular safety audits and outcome monitoring, and clear informed consent about capabilities and limitations.

Personalization Studies

Individual Differences: Growing studies focus on matching writing interventions to individual characteristics:

Personality factors: Introversion vs. extraversion may influence optimal writing approaches. Coping styles: Problem-focused vs. emotion-focused copers benefit from different techniques. Emotional expressiveness: Natural emotional expression levels predict writing intervention success. Cultural background: Adaptation needs for different cultural contexts.

Precision Medicine Approaches: Future studies aim to develop algorithms that can predict which writing interventions will work best for specific individuals based on:

Previous mental health history, current symptom patterns, personality assessments, cultural and demographic factors, and response to initial writing exercises.

STUDY LIMITATIONS AND CRITICAL CONSIDERATIONS

Understanding the limitations of current studies helps interpret findings appropriately and identify areas where caution is needed.

Current Study Gaps

High Heterogeneity: Most meta-analyses show high heterogeneity ($I^2 > 70\%$), meaning studies vary significantly in their findings. This suggests important factors that aren't yet fully understood.

Publication Bias: Like many fields, therapeutic writing studies may suffer from publication bias toward positive results. Studies showing no effect may be less likely to be published, potentially inflating apparent effectiveness.

Limited Diversity: Most study participants have been:

White, educated, Western populations, college students (easier to recruit), individuals with mild to moderate symptoms, and people comfortable with written expression.

Short-Term Follow-Up: Most studies follow participants for weeks to months rather than years, leaving questions about long-term maintenance of benefits and optimal refresher protocols.

Critical Study Needs

Long-Term Maintenance:

How do benefits maintain over years rather than months? What "booster" writing protocols help sustain improvements? How does writing effectiveness change as people age or face new life challenges?

Cultural Adaptation:

How should writing interventions be modified for different cultural contexts? What role do collective vs. individual healing approaches play? How do different languages and communication styles affect writing therapy?

Mechanism Studies:

What specific brain changes mediate therapeutic writing benefits? How do biological, psychological, and social factors interact in writing interventions? What biomarkers might predict writing intervention success?

Safety Studies:

How can we better predict who might have adverse responses to writing interventions? What are the optimal crisis detection and intervention protocols for digital platforms? How do we balance accessibility with safety in unsupervised writing interventions?

CONCLUSIONS: THE EVIDENCE-BASED FOUNDATION

The scientific evidence supports therapeutic writing as a valuable, evidence-based tool for mental health support when implemented with appropriate safeguards and realistic expectations. While effects are modest rather than miraculous, the intervention's accessibility, low cost, and scalability make it an important component of comprehensive mental health care.

Key Takeaways for Practice:

Use structured protocols based on Pennebaker's approach for maximum benefit, screen for contraindications and maintain safety protocols consistently, consider individual factors like expressiveness, culture, and current mental health status, integrate with rather than replace professional mental health treatment, and monitor outcomes using both subjective wellbeing and validated measures when possible.

The Future of Therapeutic Writing: The field stands at an exciting crossroads where traditional therapeutic writing meets technological innovation. AI-assisted platforms show remarkable promise for expanding access while maintaining safety, but human connection and professional oversight remain crucial for complex mental health challenges.

With proper implementation, mental health journaling represents a scientifically-supported intervention that can meaningfully contribute to psychological wellbeing for millions of people. The studies provide a solid foundation for the practical tools offered throughout this book, making sure that your therapeutic writing practice rests on decades of careful scientific investigation into how writing heals the mind.

APPENDIX III.
COMPLEMENTARY
APPROACHES TO MENTAL
HEALTH JOURNALING

You know how certain things naturally boost each other, like a warm drink and a good conversation? The same principle applies to mental health practices. While therapeutic journaling is powerful on its own, combining it with other evidence-based approaches can deepen your healing journey and create more comprehensive support for your emotional well-being.

Think of your mental health like a garden that thrives when multiple elements work together. Journaling provides the thoughtful reflection and self-awareness, while complementary practices offer different types of nourishment that support your overall psychological wellness. The key is finding combinations that feel natural and sustainable rather than overwhelming.

MOVEMENT AND MENTAL HEALTH: THE BODY-MIND CONNECTION

Strong connections exist between physical movement and mental health. Exercise can be as effective as medication for some types of depression, regular movement reduces anxiety and stress, and physical activity improves emotional regulation and cognitive function. When combined with therapeutic writing, movement practices can boost both physical and mental wellness.

Walking Meditation for Anxiety Relief

Walking meditation combines the anxiety-reducing benefits of gentle movement with the grounding effects of mindfulness practice. This approach is particularly helpful for people whose anxiety increases when sitting still for traditional meditation.

How to Practice Walking Meditation: Choose a quiet path 10 to 20 steps long where you won't be interrupted. Begin walking very slowly, paying attention to the sensation of each step. When your mind wanders to anxious thoughts, gently return attention to the physical sensation of walking. After 10 to 15 minutes, sit quietly and write about what you noticed during the practice.

Sarah found walking meditation transformed her relationship with anxiety: "My mind races when I try to sit still, which made traditional meditation feel impossible. But when I walk mindfully in my backyard, focusing on each step, my anxiety naturally settles. Writing afterward helps me capture insights that emerge during the peaceful state walking creates."

Integration with Therapeutic Writing: Use walking meditation as preparation before writing about anxiety-provoking topics. Practice walking meditation when writing feels too intense and you need grounding. Write about insights or observations that arise during mindful walking. Track how different walking speeds or environments affect your mental state.

Yoga and Therapeutic Writing Combinations

Yoga practice develops body awareness that can significantly boost your ability to recognize physical signals of mental health changes. The combination of movement, breath awareness, and mindfulness in yoga creates an ideal foundation for therapeutic writing.

Gentle Yoga for Mental Health: Even gentle yoga practices can reduce symptoms of anxiety, depression, and PTSD. The key is finding approaches that feel nourishing rather than demanding. Simple stretches, basic breathing exercises, and relaxation poses can provide significant mental health benefits when practiced consistently.

James discovered how yoga supported his mental health writing: "I started doing just 15 minutes of gentle stretching and breathing before my evening journal practice. The yoga helped me transition from the day's stress into a calmer state where I could access my feelings more clearly. My writing became much more honest and insightful when I prepared my body and mind this way."

Specific Combinations: Practice gentle yoga before writing sessions to create emotional and physical openness. Use yoga breathing techniques when writing brings up intense emotions. Write about body sensations and emotions that arise during yoga practice. Combine movement with processing difficult therapeutic material through alternating yoga and writing.

Exercise Journaling for Depression Management

Regular physical activity can be as effective as antidepressant medication for some people with mild to moderate depression. Combining exercise with reflective writing boosts both the physical and psychological benefits of movement.

Exercise and Mood Tracking: Writing about your physical activity and its effects on mood helps you understand what types of movement best support your mental health. This isn't about intense workouts or athletic achievement but about noticing how different forms of movement affect your emotional well-being.

Practical Exercise Journaling: Track your mood before and after different types of physical activity. Notice which forms of movement feel energizing versus draining when you're depressed. Write about barriers to exercise and strategies that help overcome them. Reflect on how movement affects sleep, appetite, and overall well-being.

Neurological Evidence for Handwriting Benefits: Studies show that handwriting activates broader neural networks than typing, engaging visual, motor, and cognitive regions simultaneously. This enhanced brain connectivity appears to be one mechanism through which writing creates therapeutic change. When combined with physical exercise, which also promotes neuroplasticity, the benefits may be amplified.

CREATIVE EXPRESSION FOR HEALING

Mental health recovery often involves rediscovering parts of yourself that may have been suppressed or forgotten during difficult periods. Creative expression provides access to emotional experiences that words alone might not reach, while also offering joy and meaning that support overall well-being.

Art Therapy Techniques with Journaling

You don't need artistic training to benefit from combining visual elements with therapeutic writing. Simple art therapy techniques can help you express emotions that feel too complex for words and access insights that purely verbal reflection might miss.

Basic Art and Writing Combinations: Draw your emotional state before writing about it, using colors and shapes rather than realistic images. Create collages about recovery goals, healing journeys, or life dreams alongside written reflections. Use simple sketches to illustrate emotions, relationships, or situations you're processing in writing. Make visual maps of support systems, triggers, or coping strategies.

Sarah found art helped her process anxiety in new ways: "I started drawing my anxiety as different colored scribbles before writing about it. Somehow seeing the anxiety on paper as these frantic red and black marks helped me understand that it was temporary energy, not a permanent part of me. This visual perspective changed how I wrote about anxious feelings and made them feel more manageable."

Integration Strategies: Alternate between drawing and writing when processing difficult emotions. Use art to explore feelings that seem too complex for words initially. Create visual representations of mental health goals and write about steps toward achieving them. Draw your support system and reflect on relationships through writing.

Music and Mental Health Reflection

Music has unique power to access and evoke emotions, making it a valuable companion to therapeutic writing. Music can improve mood, reduce anxiety, and boost emotional processing when used thoughtfully in mental health practices.

Music-Enhanced Writing Practices: Create playlists that support different types of reflection: calming music for anxiety processing, uplifting songs for depression recovery, or instrumental music for focused writing. Write about songs that resonate with your mental health experience. Use lyrics as prompts for personal reflection. Notice how different types of music affect your ability to access emotions.

James discovered music opened emotional doors: "I made a playlist of songs that seemed to understand my depression better than I did. Listening to these songs before writing helped me access feelings I couldn't reach any other way. Sometimes I'd write about why certain lyrics resonated with me, which led to insights about my own experience I wouldn't have found otherwise."

Therapeutic Music Guidelines: Choose music that supports rather than intensifies difficult emotions when you're vulnerable. Use calming or neutral music when processing trauma or intense anxiety. Notice whether certain songs trigger negative emotional spirals and avoid them during therapeutic writing. Experiment with instrumental music if lyrics feel distracting during reflection.

Poetry for Emotional Processing

Poetic language can capture emotional experiences that prose cannot adequately express. You don't need to be a poet to benefit from exploring feelings through imagery, metaphor, and rhythm. Simple poetic exercises can unlock new understanding and provide emotional relief.

Accessible Poetry Techniques: Write about emotions using only sensory language (what you see, hear, feel, taste, smell). Create simple metaphors for your mental health experience (depression is like..., anxiety feels like...). Use repetitive phrases to explore themes (I am learning..., I used to think..., Now I know...). Write letters to your emotions, treating them as separate entities you can dialogue with.

Poetry and Mental Health Benefits: Poetry often requires fewer words than prose, making it accessible during low-energy periods. Metaphorical language can provide safe distance from overwhelming emotions. Rhythm and repetition can be soothing and grounding. Creative expression often brings unexpected joy even while processing difficult topics.

MINDFULNESS PRACTICES THAT BOOST THERAPEUTIC WRITING

Mindfulness, the practice of paying attention to the present moment without judgment, significantly boosts therapeutic writing by increasing emotional awareness, reducing reactivity to difficult feelings, and creating space for insights to emerge naturally.

Meditation and Therapeutic Writing

Brief meditation before writing sessions can help you access deeper emotional awareness while reducing mental chatter that might interfere with honest reflection. Even five minutes of simple breathing practice can create valuable space for therapeutic exploration.

Simple Pre-Writing Meditation: Sit comfortably and focus on your breath for 3 to 5 minutes. Notice thoughts and feelings without trying to change them. When your attention wanders, gently return to breathing. After meditation, begin writing while maintaining the same gentle, non-judgmental awareness.

Mindful Writing Practice: Pay attention to the physical sensation of writing, how the pen feels in your hand, the sound it makes on paper, the formation of letters and words. Notice thoughts and feelings as they arise during writing without immediately judging them as good or bad. Stay present with whatever emotional material emerges, breathing through difficult moments.

Sarah learned to combine mindfulness with writing: "I used to rush into journaling and then get overwhelmed by whatever emotions came up. When I started taking a few minutes to breathe and center myself first, my writing became much more peaceful and insightful. I could stay present with difficult feelings instead of getting swept away by them."

Body Awareness for Trauma Recovery

For people with trauma histories, developing gentle body awareness through mindfulness can support therapeutic writing by helping you recognize when you're approaching emotional limits and need to slow down or seek additional support.

Gentle Body Scanning: Before writing, spend a few minutes noticing physical sensations throughout your body. Start with your feet and slowly move your attention up through your legs, torso, arms, and head. Notice areas of tension, relaxation, warmth, coolness, or any other sensations without trying to change them.

Window of Tolerance Awareness: Learn to recognize your "window of tolerance," the zone where you feel alert but not overwhelmed, calm but not numb. When writing begins to push you outside this window (feeling either overwhelmed or disconnected), use body awareness to guide you back to emotional balance.

Safety Protocols for Trauma Writing: Never write about trauma when you're already feeling overwhelmed or dysregulated. Use grounding techniques if writing activates trauma responses. Keep writing sessions short (15-20 minutes maximum) when processing traumatic material. Have professional support available for trauma-focused writing.

James found body awareness crucial for safe trauma processing: "I learned to check in with my body before and during writing about difficult experiences. When I noticed my shoulders getting tight or my breathing becoming shallow, I'd take a break and do some grounding exercises. This body awareness helped me process trauma at a pace my nervous system could handle."

Present Moment Practice for Anxiety

Anxiety often involves worry about future events that may never happen or rumination about past events that cannot be changed. Mindfulness practices that anchor attention in the present moment can provide relief from anxious thinking patterns and create space for more balanced perspective.

Grounding Techniques for Anxious Writing: Use the 5-4-3-2-1 technique before writing when anxiety is present: notice 5 things you can see, 4 things you can touch, 3 things you can hear, 2 things you can smell, and 1 thing you can taste. Practice "noting" anxious thoughts without engaging with their content ("I notice worry about tomorrow"). Return attention to present-moment sensations when writing becomes future-focused.

Present-Moment Writing Prompts: What do you notice in your immediate environment right now? How does your body feel in this moment? What emotions are present without any story about why they're there? What sounds, smells, or physical sensations can you observe?

THERAPEUTIC RITUAL AND RHYTHM

Creating simple rituals around your mental health practice can make therapeutic writing feel more meaningful and sustainable. Rituals help signal to your mind that this is important time for healing and self-care.

Creating Sacred Healing Space

Your writing environment significantly affects the quality of your therapeutic practice. Creating a space that feels safe, private, and nurturing supports deeper reflection and emotional processing.

Elements of Therapeutic Writing Space: Choose a location where you won't be interrupted or observed. Make sure you have comfortable seating and good lighting for extended writing. Keep supplies (journal, pen, tissues, water) easily accessible. Consider adding elements that support calm focus: candles, plants, meaningful objects, or calming scents.

Sarah created ritual around her writing space: "I have this special corner in my bedroom with a comfortable chair, good lamp, and a small table for my journal and tea. When I sit in that space, my mind automatically shifts into a more reflective mode. The physical environment helps signal that this is healing time, separate from the rest of my day."

Digital vs. Physical Spaces: While handwriting offers neurological advantages, some people need to use digital tools for accessibility reasons. If writing digitally, create virtual ritual: special music, lighting, or other environmental cues that signal therapeutic writing time.

Timing Your Mental Health Practice

Different times of day can be optimal for different types of mental health reflection. Understanding your natural rhythms helps you choose timing that supports rather than stresses your therapeutic practice.

Morning Writing Benefits: Accessing emotions and insights before daily stress accumulates. Processing dreams and unconscious material that surfaces during sleep. Setting intentions for mental health support throughout the day. Clearing emotional material before engaging with work or relationship demands.

Evening Writing Benefits: Reflecting on and integrating the day's emotional experiences. Processing challenges while they're still fresh in memory. Releasing stress and worry before sleep. Preparing for restorative rest through emotional clearing.

James found his optimal timing through experimentation: "I tried morning writing for weeks but always felt rushed and stressed about getting to work. When I switched to evening reflection, everything changed. I could take my time processing the day's emotions without worrying about what came next. My sleep improved because I wasn't carrying unprocessed stress to bed."

Seasonal Mental Health Awareness

Your mental health naturally fluctuates with seasons, life transitions, and anniversary dates of significant events. Incorporating awareness of these rhythms into your therapeutic writing practice helps you prepare for and navigate predictable challenges.

Seasonal Adjustments: Notice how different seasons affect your mood, energy, and mental health needs. Adjust writing topics and frequency based on seasonal mental health patterns. Use seasonal transitions as prompts for deeper reflection about growth and change. Plan additional support during seasons that consistently challenge your mental health.

Anniversary Reactions: Be aware that anniversary dates of trauma, loss, or other significant events can trigger emotional responses even when you're not consciously thinking about them. Use therapeutic writing to process anniversary reactions with extra gentleness and professional support when needed.

WORKING WITH MENTAL HEALTH DREAMS

Dreams often provide access to emotional material and unconscious wisdom that can boost therapeutic writing. While dream interpretation isn't necessary, paying attention to dreams can enrich your understanding of your mental health patterns and needs.

Dream Journaling for Processing

Keep a notebook by your bed to capture dreams before they fade from memory. Write dreams in present tense as if they're happening now. Include emotions, colors, sensations, and atmosphere, not just events. Notice recurring themes, characters, or settings that might relate to your waking mental health concerns.

Integration with Therapeutic Writing: Use dream imagery as metaphors for exploring waking life challenges. Write dialogues with dream figures to access different perspectives. Notice correlations between dream content and mental health patterns.

Explore emotions from dreams that might be suppressed during waking hours.

Sarah found dreams offered unexpected insights: "I kept having these dreams about being lost in mazes during a particularly anxious period. When I wrote about these dreams, I realized the maze represented how overwhelmed I felt by all my options and decisions. This insight helped me understand that my anxiety wasn't about external dangers but about feeling confused about direction in my life."

Active Imagination Techniques

Active imagination involves consciously engaging with dream imagery or spontaneous mental images to explore their meaning and emotional significance. This technique, developed by Carl Jung, can be safely adapted for mental health journaling.

Simple Active Imagination: Choose a dream image or spontaneous mental image that feels significant. In your journal, have a written conversation with this image, asking what it represents or what it wants you to know. Write from the image's perspective, letting it speak back to you. Notice what insights or emotions emerge through this imaginal dialogue.

Safety Considerations: Use active imagination only with benign or neutral images, not frightening or overwhelming ones. Keep sessions brief (10-15 minutes) to avoid becoming lost in fantasy. Ground yourself in present-moment reality before and after active imagination exercises. Seek professional guidance if imaginal work brings up intense trauma material.

GROUP MENTAL HEALTH PRACTICE

While therapeutic writing is often a solitary practice, sharing aspects of your journey with others can provide perspective, reduce isolation, and offer encouragement during challenging periods. The key is maintaining appropriate boundaries about what to share while still benefiting from community support.

Therapeutic Writing Circles

Many communities offer writing groups specifically designed for people working on mental health recovery. These groups typically focus on the therapeutic benefits of writing rather than literary critique, providing safe spaces to explore emotional topics through structured writing exercises.

What to Look for in Therapeutic Writing Groups: Facilitators with mental health training or supervision from professionals. Clear guidelines about confidentiality and emotional safety. Focus on personal healing rather than writing quality or performance. Integration with professional mental health resources in the community. Appropriate crisis intervention protocols if participants become overwhelmed.

James found community through a therapeutic writing group: "I was hesitant to share anything about my mental health struggles, but the writing group provided this middle ground where I could be around others working on similar challenges without having to reveal private details. Just being in the presence of other people committed to healing felt supportive."

Boundaries and Privacy: You never need to share journal content that feels too private or vulnerable. Many groups focus on writing exercises done in the moment rather than sharing previous personal writing. Consider what level of sharing feels safe and supportive rather than exposing or overwhelming.

Mental Health Accountability Partners

Having a journaling buddy can help maintain your therapeutic writing practice while providing mutual support for mental health goals. This works best when both people understand appropriate boundaries and limitations.

Effective Accountability Partnerships: Check in regularly about maintaining writing practice without sharing private content. Support each other's commitment to self-care and professional treatment when needed. Share insights about what helps maintain consistent therapeutic writing without requiring detailed personal disclosure. Celebrate progress and provide encouragement during difficult periods.

What Accountability Partners Should NOT Do: Provide therapy or professional mental health advice. Pressure each other to share private journal content. Take responsibility for each other's mental health or crisis intervention. Replace professional treatment with peer support.

Sarah found accountability helpful: "My friend and I text each other a few times a week just to check that we're both keeping up with our writing practice. We don't share what we write about, but knowing someone else cares about my commitment to self-care helps me prioritize it even when life gets busy."

INTEGRATION WITH PROFESSIONAL TREATMENT

Therapeutic writing can significantly boost professional mental health treatment when integrated thoughtfully and with appropriate professional guidance. The key is understanding how writing can support rather than replace professional care.

Journaling Between Therapy Sessions

Many therapists welcome therapeutic writing as homework between appointments. Your journal entries can provide valuable information about patterns, triggers, and progress that might not be apparent during brief therapy sessions.

Effective Integration Strategies: Share relevant insights from your writing practice during therapy sessions. Use prompts to prepare for therapy by clarifying what you want to discuss.

Write about therapy sessions afterward to integrate new perspectives and insights. Track medication effects, side effects, and mood changes through therapeutic writing.

Boundaries with Therapists: Not all journal content needs to be shared with your therapist. Maintain areas of privacy while still benefiting from professional support. Focus on sharing patterns and insights rather than reading entire journal entries during sessions. Ask your therapist about specific writing exercises that might support your treatment goals.

Medication Tracking Through Writing

If you take psychiatric medications, therapeutic writing can help you and your prescribing provider make informed decisions about dosage, timing, and medication changes through careful tracking of effects and side effects.

Medication Journaling: Track your mood, energy, sleep, and other relevant symptoms daily. Note timing of medication doses and any missed doses. Record side effects and their impact on daily functioning. Write about your overall experience with medication treatment, including hopes, fears, and questions.

James found medication tracking invaluable: "Writing about my daily experience with antidepressants helped my psychiatrist understand how the medication was affecting me beyond just the basic rating scales we used during appointments. My journal showed patterns in when side effects occurred and how the medication interacted with stress, sleep, and other factors."

Treatment Goal Journaling

Therapeutic writing can help you maintain motivation and track progress toward therapy goals while providing space to explore ambivalence or challenges that arise during treatment.

Goal-Focused Writing: Write about your hopes and expectations for mental health treatment. Track specific goals and gradual progress toward achieving them. Explore obstacles or resistance that arise during treatment. Celebrate small victories and learning experiences along the way.

Collaboration with Treatment Providers: Discuss your writing practice with your treatment team to make sure it supports rather than conflicts with professional goals. Share pattern recognition from your journaling that might inform treatment planning. Use writing to practice therapeutic techniques between professional sessions.

CREATING YOUR PERSONALIZED MENTAL HEALTH PRACTICE

The most effective mental health practices are those that feel natural, sustainable, and authentically yours. While evidence-based approaches provide valuable guidance, your personal preferences, cultural background, and individual needs should ultimately shape how you integrate different practices.

Sarah reflects on developing her integrated practice: "I started by trying everything at once, thinking more practices would create faster healing. That approach felt overwhelming and unsustainable. When I learned to add one element at a time and really notice how each addition affected my mental health, I could create a practice that genuinely supported my well-being instead of adding stress to my life."

James found his way through gentle experimentation: "I began with just therapeutic journaling and slowly added other elements as I felt ready. First yoga, then mindfulness meditation, eventually creative expression through music. Building my practice gradually helped me understand what each element contributed and how they worked together to support my mental health."

Guidelines for Integration: Start with one primary practice (like therapeutic journaling) and develop consistency before adding other elements. Add new practices one at a time, giving yourself several weeks to notice their effects. Pay attention to what feels nourishing versus what feels burdensome. Adjust or eliminate practices that don't serve your mental health goals.

Remember that your practice will evolve as you do. What supports your mental health during crisis periods might be different from what you need during stable times. Seasonal changes, life transitions, and personal growth all affect what practices feel most helpful. Trust your developing wisdom about what serves your mental health best.

THE ART OF SUSTAINABLE MENTAL HEALTH PRACTICE

Creating a sustainable mental health practice is like tending a garden. It requires consistent attention but not constant intensity. The goal is developing approaches that support your well-being over time rather than creating additional stress or pressure in your life.

Principles of Sustainability: Choose practices that feel nurturing rather than demanding. Adapt your practice to your current mental health state and life circumstances. Focus on consistency over perfection. Small regular efforts create more benefit than sporadic intensive practices. Build flexibility into your routine to accommodate life's natural changes and challenges.

Your complementary practices should feel like gentle additions to your therapeutic writing rather than obligations you must fulfill. Let your intuition guide you toward approaches that resonate with your personality, cultural background, and current needs. The most powerful mental health practice is the one you can maintain with kindness toward yourself.

As you explore these complementary approaches, remember that therapeutic writing remains the foundation that can support and be supported by other mental health practices. Each element you add should boost rather than complicate your relationship with yourself and your healing journey.

Trust that you have the wisdom to create a mental health practice that serves your unique needs while drawing from the evidence-based approaches that have helped millions of people find greater peace, resilience, and well-being. Your journey toward mental wellness is as individual as you are, and these tools are here to support whatever path feels authentic and healing for you.

APPENDIX IV. EVIDENCE-BASED SAFETY FOUNDATION

You know how a well-designed garden includes both beautiful plants and protective barriers that keep everything thriving safely? Mental health journaling requires the same thoughtful approach to safety. While therapeutic writing offers tremendous benefits for emotional well-being, it also requires careful attention to when it's helpful and when professional support is needed instead.

This appendix provides the evidence-based safety foundation that underlies all the prompts and practices in this book. Think of it as your comprehensive guide for maintaining both the therapeutic benefits and safety of your mental health journaling practice.

PRE-SCREENING ASSESSMENT: UNDERSTANDING YOUR STARTING POINT

Before beginning any therapeutic writing practice, it's important to honestly assess whether self-guided journaling is appropriate for your current situation. This isn't about excluding people from healing opportunities but making sure that everyone gets the right type of support for their specific needs.

Emotional Expressiveness Evaluation

People vary significantly in their natural comfort with identifying and expressing emotions. Those with high emotional expressiveness typically benefit more from traditional expressive writing approaches, while others might need adapted techniques or professional support.

Assess Your Emotional Expressiveness: Do you typically notice and can identify specific emotions (sad, frustrated, excited) rather than general states (good, bad, stressed)? When friends ask how you're feeling, do you usually have ready access to that information? Can you describe emotional experiences in detail when you choose to? Do you feel comfortable expressing emotions verbally or in writing?

If you answered "no" to most of these questions, you might have alexithymia (difficulty identifying emotions), which can make standard expressive writing frustrating or unhelpful. This doesn't mean writing can't support your mental health, but you might benefit from starting with more structured, cognitive-focused prompts or working with a therapist who understands alexithymia.

Sarah discovered this about herself: "I realized I'd been frustrated with journaling because I kept trying to write about feelings I couldn't actually identify. When I learned that some people need to start with thoughts and behaviors before accessing emotions, I could adjust my approach and actually benefit from the practice."

Recent Trauma History: The Six-Month Rule

Studies consistently show that writing about trauma within six months of the traumatic event can potentially retraumatize rather than heal. This doesn't mean you can't write at all during this period, but trauma-focused writing should be conducted with professional supervision.

Recent Trauma Considerations: Have you experienced any traumatic events (accidents, violence, sudden loss, medical trauma) within the past six months? Are you still experiencing acute stress symptoms like intrusive thoughts, nightmares, or emotional numbness related to recent trauma? Do you find yourself avoiding reminders of recent difficult experiences? Are you currently in crisis mode or survival mode from recent events?

If you answered "yes" to these questions, focus on present-moment writing rather than trauma processing. Use daily foundation prompts that keep you grounded in current experience. Seek professional trauma-informed therapy for processing recent traumatic experiences. Consider this book's situational prompts for anxiety or stress rather than deeper trauma-focused work.

James learned this lesson: "I started trying to write about my divorce immediately after it happened, thinking it would help me process. Instead, it just stirred up all the pain without helping me make sense of it. When I waited and worked with a therapist first, writing eventually became a helpful part of my healing, but not while everything was still so raw."

Current Mental Health Status Assessment

Your current mental health status significantly influences whether self-guided therapeutic writing is appropriate and what safety measures you need. This assessment helps you understand what level of support would best serve your healing journey.

Current Mental Health Evaluation: Are you currently in crisis or experiencing thoughts of self-harm or suicide? Do you have severe symptoms that significantly interfere with daily functioning (work, relationships, self-care)? Are you experiencing psychosis, severe dissociation, or other symptoms that affect your connection to reality? Do you have adequate professional mental health support for your current needs?

Current crisis or severe symptoms require immediate professional intervention rather than self-guided writing approaches. Moderate symptoms often benefit from therapeutic writing combined with professional support. Mild symptoms or maintenance periods can safely include self-guided writing with appropriate safety protocols.

Cultural and Language Considerations

Most therapeutic writing studies have been conducted with Western, English-speaking populations where individual emotional expression is culturally encouraged. If you come from different cultural backgrounds, you might need to adapt approaches to feel authentic and helpful.

Cultural Assessment Questions: Does your cultural background emphasize individual emotional expression or collective well-being? What are the norms in your culture around sharing personal struggles or seeking help? Do you feel comfortable writing in your first language about emotional topics? Would family or community members support your engagement in therapeutic writing?

Adaptation might involve writing in your native language if that feels more emotionally accessible, incorporating cultural values around family or community in your reflection, seeking therapeutic writing approaches designed for your cultural background, or finding professional support from culturally informed mental health providers.

CONTRAINDICATIONS AND RED FLAGS: WHEN TO SEEK PROFESSIONAL HELP

Studies identify specific situations where unsupervised therapeutic writing can be problematic or insufficient for mental health needs. Understanding these contraindications protects your well-being and helps you make informed decisions about when to seek professional support.

Absolute Contraindications

Active Psychosis Without Professional Supervision: If you're experiencing hallucinations, delusions, or significant disconnection from reality, therapeutic writing should only be conducted under professional supervision. Psychotic symptoms can make it difficult to distinguish between thoughts, feelings, and reality, which is necessary for safe therapeutic writing.

Alexithymia (Severe Difficulty Identifying Emotions): People with alexithymia often find traditional expressive writing frustrating because they can't access the emotional material that these approaches require. This can lead to increased distress rather than relief. If you have alexithymia, consider cognitive-focused writing approaches or professional support that addresses this condition specifically.

Acute Trauma Within Six Months: Recent trauma requires specialized professional intervention rather than self-guided writing approaches. Writing about acute trauma without proper support can potentially retraumatize by overwhelming your emotional regulation capacity.

Relative Contraindications

Low Emotional Expressiveness: If you naturally have difficulty accessing or expressing emotions, standard expressive writing approaches might feel forced or unhelpful. You might benefit more from structured, cognitive-focused prompts or professional guidance in developing emotional awareness gradually.

High Dissociation Tendency: People prone to dissociative responses (feeling disconnected from thoughts, feelings, or physical sensations) need specialized approaches to therapeutic writing that include grounding and present-moment awareness techniques.

Compulsive Behaviors Around Writing: If you find yourself unable to control or limit writing sessions, or if writing becomes a compulsive behavior you use to avoid other life activities, professional support can help address underlying issues that drive compulsive responses.

Warning Signs Requiring Immediate Professional Intervention

During Writing Sessions: Stop writing and seek professional help if you experience ongoing distress lasting more than two hours after writing sessions, increased symptoms of depression or anxiety that worsen after writing, overwhelming emotions that feel completely out of control, or panic attacks or severe anxiety triggered by writing.

Pattern Recognition: Seek professional consultation if you notice writing sessions consistently make you feel worse rather than better, you're unable to limit writing time or frequency despite negative consequences, writing becomes a way to avoid necessary life activities or relationships, or you find yourself writing about self-harm or suicide.

Crisis Situations: Seek immediate professional help (call 911, go to emergency room, or call crisis hotline) if you experience thoughts of self-harm or suicide, plans to hurt yourself or others, complete loss of connection to reality, or severe symptoms that interfere with basic functioning.

SAFETY PROTOCOLS DURING PRACTICE

Even when therapeutic writing is appropriate for your situation, following evidence-based safety protocols protects your well-being and maximizes the therapeutic benefits of your practice.

Time Limits and Session Structure

Evidence-Based Time Guidelines: Limit writing sessions to 20 minutes maximum to prevent emotional overwhelm. Take breaks every 15 minutes during longer reflection periods to check in with your emotional state. Allow at least 10 minutes after writing for cooldown and grounding before returning to daily activities.

Session Spacing: Space intensive writing sessions at least 24 hours apart to allow time for emotional processing. Avoid writing about difficult topics when you're already emotionally overwhelmed or in crisis. Schedule writing during times when you have adequate time and space for processing afterward.

Sarah learned the importance of time limits: "I used to think longer writing sessions would be more beneficial, but I discovered that after about 20 minutes, I'd start spiraling instead of processing. Setting a timer helped me stay within therapeutic limits and actually get more benefit from shorter, focused sessions."

Cooldown and Grounding Techniques

Post-Writing Grounding: After each writing session, spend 5 to 10 minutes returning your attention to the present moment using grounding techniques. Practice deep breathing to regulate your nervous system. Engage in physical movement to help integrate emotional processing. Do something nurturing for yourself like drinking tea, listening to music, or stepping outside.

Effective Grounding Techniques: Use the 5-4-3-2-1 technique: notice 5 things you can see, 4 things you can touch, 3 things you can hear, 2 things you can smell, and 1 thing you can taste. Practice progressive muscle relaxation by tensing and releasing different muscle groups. Focus on your breath with simple counting: inhale for 4, hold for 4, exhale for 6.

James found grounding essential: "I learned that writing sessions could leave me feeling emotionally raw, especially early in my practice. Taking time to ground myself afterward helped me transition back to daily life without carrying intense emotions with me all day."

Emergency Contact Procedures

Immediate Support Resources: Keep crisis hotline numbers easily accessible in your writing space and programmed into your phone. Have contact information for your mental health providers if you're currently in treatment. Identify trusted friends or family members who could provide support if needed. Know the location and contact information for your nearest emergency mental health services.

Crisis Contact Information: National Suicide Prevention Lifeline: 988, Crisis Text Line: Text HOME to 741741, National Alliance on Mental Illness (NAMI): 1-800-950-NAMI, or call 911 for immediate emergency assistance.

Professional Backup Requirements

When Professional Backup Is Essential: If you're currently managing moderate to severe mental health symptoms, maintain ongoing professional support even while using self-guided writing. If you have a history of trauma, make sure you have access to trauma-informed therapists when needed. If you're taking psychiatric medications, maintain regular contact with your prescribing provider.

Collaboration with Existing Providers: Discuss your therapeutic writing practice with current mental health providers to make sure it complements your treatment. Share relevant insights from your writing practice that might inform professional treatment. Ask about specific writing exercises that might support your treatment goals.

MONITORING AND OUTCOME TRACKING

Regular monitoring of your mental health and response to therapeutic writing helps make sure the practice continues to serve your well-being and alerts you to when adjustments or professional support might be needed.

Evidence-Based Assessment Tools

Simple Self-Monitoring: Track your mood before and after writing sessions using a simple 1-10 scale. Notice patterns in what types of writing help versus what makes you feel worse. Monitor changes in sleep, appetite, energy, and daily functioning. Keep track of your overall life satisfaction and stress levels over time.

Standardized Assessment Tools: Consider using validated measures like the PHQ-9 for depression symptoms or GAD-7 for anxiety symptoms monthly to track changes over time. These tools provide objective measures that can help you and any professional providers understand your progress.

Red Flag Behavioral Indicators: Watch for increasing isolation or withdrawal from relationships, declining performance at work or school, changes in sleep patterns or appetite, increased substance use or other unhealthy coping behaviors, or loss of interest in activities you usually enjoy.

Sarah found tracking valuable: "I started keeping simple notes about my mood before and after writing sessions. This helped me realize that certain types of prompts consistently helped my anxiety while others sometimes made it worse. Understanding these patterns helped me choose writing approaches that actually supported my mental health."

Progress Tracking Methods

Positive Indicators: Look for increased emotional awareness and vocabulary, better recognition of your own patterns and triggers, improved ability to self-soothe during difficult emotions, enhanced problem-solving and decision-making skills, and stronger sense of self-compassion and acceptance.

Concerning Patterns: Be alert to writing sessions that consistently increase distress, avoidance of daily responsibilities to write, increased rumination or obsessive thinking, deteriorating relationships or work performance, or loss of perspective about problems or life circumstances.

When to Modify or Discontinue Practice

Modifications That Might Help: Reduce writing frequency if sessions feel overwhelming, focus on less emotionally charged topics, add more structure through specific prompts, increase grounding and self-care around writing sessions, or seek professional guidance for adapting your approach.

When to Discontinue: Stop therapeutic writing if it consistently worsens your mental health symptoms, if you develop compulsive writing behaviors you can't control, if writing becomes a way to avoid necessary treatment or life activities, or if you're experiencing thoughts of self-harm related to writing practice.

James learned to adjust his practice: "During a particularly stressful period, I noticed my writing sessions were making my anxiety worse instead of better. I took a break for a few weeks and then returned with shorter, more structured sessions that felt more manageable. Learning to modify my practice based on my current needs was crucial for long-term sustainability."

PROFESSIONAL INTEGRATION GUIDELINES

Understanding how to effectively integrate therapeutic writing with professional mental health care boosts both your self-guided practice and any professional treatment you receive.

When to Recommend Professional Help

Clear Indicators for Professional Support: Seek professional help if you experience ongoing symptoms that interfere with daily functioning, thoughts of self-harm or suicide, symptoms that don't improve with self-care approaches including writing, or trauma that needs specialized treatment approaches.

Types of Professional Support: Individual therapy can provide personalized guidance and support for mental health challenges. Psychiatry offers medication evaluation and management when appropriate. Support groups provide community and shared experiences with others facing similar challenges. Specialized programs address specific conditions like trauma, eating disorders, or substance use.

Collaboration with Existing Treatment Providers

Effective Collaboration Strategies: Share relevant insights from your writing practice during therapy sessions without feeling pressured to share private journal content. Ask your therapist about specific writing exercises that might support your treatment goals. Use writing to prepare for therapy sessions by clarifying what you want to discuss. Track medication effects and therapy progress through structured writing.

Boundaries and Privacy: Remember that not all journal content needs to be shared with professional providers. Focus on sharing patterns and insights rather than detailed personal writing.

Maintain appropriate boundaries about what feels private versus what would be helpful to share.

Documentation and Communication Protocols

Helpful Documentation: Keep records of which writing approaches help versus hinder your mental health. Track patterns in your responses to different types of prompts. Note any concerning symptoms or responses that arise during writing practice. Document progress toward mental health goals over time.

Communication with Providers: Be honest about your therapeutic writing practice so providers can offer appropriate guidance. Ask questions about how writing can best support your specific treatment goals. Report any concerning responses to writing so adjustments can be made as needed.

Ethical Considerations for Self-Guided vs. Supervised Practice

Self-Guided Practice Appropriateness: Self-guided therapeutic writing is most appropriate for people with mild to moderate symptoms who have adequate coping skills and social support. It works well for maintenance periods between therapy or as an adjunct to professional treatment. It's helpful for people who want to boost their self-awareness and emotional regulation skills.

When Supervision Is Necessary: Professional supervision is essential for severe mental health symptoms, recent trauma processing, people with limited emotional awareness or coping skills, or anyone experiencing thoughts of self-harm or suicide.

Informed Decision-Making: Understanding these guidelines helps you make informed decisions about when self-guided writing is appropriate and when professional support would better serve your mental health needs. The goal is making sure everyone receives the right level of care for their specific situation.

CREATING YOUR PERSONAL SAFETY PLAN

Your personal safety plan integrates all these guidelines into a practical system that protects your well-being while supporting your therapeutic writing practice.

Before You Begin Writing: Assess your current emotional state and choose appropriate prompts accordingly. Make sure you have adequate time and privacy for both writing and post-session processing. Have grounding techniques and support resources easily accessible. Set clear time limits for your writing session.

During Writing Sessions: Monitor your emotional state and take breaks if you become overwhelmed. Use grounding techniques if you feel disconnected or overly activated. Stop writing if you experience thoughts of self-harm or severe distress. Remember that you can always return to a topic when you feel more resourced.

After Writing Sessions: Take time to ground yourself and transition back to daily activities. Notice how the writing session affected your mood and overall state. Practice self-care activities that support your well-being. Reach out for support if you're feeling overwhelmed or need to process the session with someone else.

Long-Term Monitoring: Regularly assess whether your writing practice continues to support your mental health goals. Adjust your approach based on what you learn about your responses to different techniques. Seek professional consultation when you notice concerning patterns or need additional support.

Remember that these safety guidelines exist to protect and support your healing journey, not to create barriers to your growth. The goal is making sure that therapeutic writing remains a positive, beneficial practice that boosts rather than complicates your mental health and well-being.

Your safety and healing matter most. Trust your instincts about what feels right for your mental health journey, and don't hesitate to seek professional support whenever you feel it would be helpful. The combination of evidence-based self-care tools and professional mental health support, when needed, provides the strongest foundation for lasting mental wellness.

NOTE FROM THE AUTHOR

Dear Reader,

Thank you for investing your valuable time in this book. I trust that these insights and principles have provided you with practical tools for your personal, professional, or spiritual journey.

Your engagement with this material means a great deal, and I'd be grateful if you'd consider sharing your experience with others. Would you take a moment to leave an honest review? Your feedback not only helps others discover these resources but also contributes to our collective growth and learning.

Your insights can be shared on any of these platforms:

📖 Amazon 　 Goodreads

Want to stay connected? I'd love to keep you updated on new releases and exclusive content:

• Subscribe to weekly insights: Journalinginsights.com

With appreciation for your commitment to growth,

Richard French

ABOUT THE AUTHOR

Richard French, a pioneering technology leader and entrepreneur, brings his wealth of experience in innovation and personal growth to the realm of journaling. As a driving force behind several successful technology companies, Richard has consistently demonstrated the power of self-reflection and clear goal-setting in achieving remarkable business transformations.

With a career spanning software, AI, and global business leadership, Richard has guided organizations from startup stage to multi-million dollar enterprises. His philosophy that "people work with us, not for us" underlies his approach to personal development and team building.

A mathematics graduate and GT race car driver, Richard combines analytical thinking with a passion for pushing boundaries. In "Write Your Way," he applies his unique perspective on goal achievement and self-expression, offering readers a roadmap to personal transformation drawn from his experiences in the fast-paced worlds of technology and motorsports.

Richard's insights, honed through years of leading innovation and speaking at industry conferences, now guide readers on their journey of self-discovery through the power of journaling.

www.ingramcontent.com/pod-product-compliance
Lightning Source LLC
Chambersburg PA
CBHW071238130626
46556CB00003B/1070